Histamine Lifehacks

Histamine in Balance: From Biological Roles to Managing Histamine Intolerance

Debbie Moon, MSc

Case studies by Dr. Ibby Omole, ND, MSA

Table of Contents

About the Authors

Debbie Moon is the founder of Genetic Lifehacks (www.GeneticLifehacks.com). At Genetic Lifehacks, Debbie Moon focuses on sharing current health research, with an emphasis on explaining how genetic variants influence health and wellness.

Debbie has a BS in engineering and a Master of Science in Biological Science. Her passion is making current research accessible and understandable for everyone. She applies an engineering mindset to current genetics and health research, tying together the concepts to present a fuller picture with personalized applications. Debbie currently lives in Montana, enjoying the beautiful mountains and wide-open spaces.

Dr. Ibby Omole (www.driomole.com) is a naturopathic doctor who uses a Lifestyle Medicine approach that focuses on helping individuals gain clarity about their health by focusing on nutrition, physical movement, stress management, sleep, and social connection using an evidence-based method. Her clinical areas of expertise are digestive health (IBS/SIBO), fertility, pelvic health conditions, and genetic analysis. She has worked in integrative clinics in the United States and Canada. She previously held a core faculty position at CCNM - Boucher campus where she was involved in curriculum development and clinical training of naturopathic students.

Dr. Omole is an avid outdoors enthusiast and foodie. She can often be found enjoying the great Canadian outdoors winter or summer with her two boys.

Disclaimer: Everything in this book is for educational and informational purposes and not intended as medical advice. Please consult your doctor for medical advice.

Introduction

Are you constantly clearing your throat because of sinus drainage after you eat? Do you get periodic itching, hives, or rashes that come and go? What about migraines, irritability, anxiety, brain fog? Stomach ailments and intestinal issues? Waking up at 3 am?

These seemingly unrelated symptoms can be due to an excess level of histamine.

Classified as a biogenic amine, histamine is a molecule that plays many roles in the body. Histamine's many functions include:

- causes allergic reactions
- acts within our immune defense system
- dilates blood vessels (vasodilatation)
- acts as a neurotransmitter
- works as a signaling molecule in the stomach to release acid

While most of us think of histamine only during allergy season, histamine is a vital part of how your body works. The key is that you want the right amount—not too much!

Why Histamine Lifehacks?

There are a lot of people dealing with histamine-related symptoms who do not know that high histamine levels are at the root of their issues. Rather than understanding and resolving the root causes, they often end up cycling through antihistamines, heartburn medications, gut healing protocols, topical creams, and migraine drugs.

My goal is to help people understand the underlying physiology that drives their symptoms. I'm going to explain the current research on histamine, covering the diverse ways that it affects your body.

Histamine Lifehacks refers to a broadly encompassing picture that includes solutions for high histamine levels from multiple sources.

Many focus solely on histamine intolerance, but the scientific research presents a much bigger story—one of multiple ways that an excess of histamine can occur. This story goes beyond a basic food intolerance, as it encompasses various factors like our diet and chemical exposure. So whether you have histamine intolerance, high gut histamine production, or histamine-related symptoms from mast cell activation, this book is for you.

The "Lifehacks" part of Histamine Lifehacks takes the scientific research one step further to cover lifestyle changes, dietary considerations, and natural supplement solutions.

My goal is to present the science, explain the research studies, and provide options for solutions that you can explore. There is no one-size-fits-all protocol here. Everyone has a unique exposure to different substances, unique reactions of their body, and a unique composition of the gut microbiome. You decide what works best for you, as a unique individual, and then talk with your doctor if you need medical advice.

Research studies can show us statistics, mechanisms of action, and causation. While this is all great information to understand, in reality, life is messy, and people are unique. So, keep in mind that high histamine may only be part of the picture for your unique situation.

Case Studies for Clarity

In many chapters of this book, you will find case studies by Dr. Ibby Omole, a naturopathic physician with more than two decades of experience in treating patients with a holistic approach. The case studies will give you a glimpse into how a naturopathic physician sees and treats histamine-related issues.

You'll find that the case studies don't fit neatly into categories. This is because histamine-related health issues cross many categories, and people are all unique in their exposure, lifestyle, and genetic susceptibility. You'll see that lowering high histamine levels can help in a variety of ways, but that histamine is only part of the bigger health picture for many people.

To protect patient privacy, we fictionalize all names and personal details.

Overview of Chapters

Chapter 1: Histamine Overload - Introduces the concept of histamine intolerance and explores the various symptoms associated with high histamine levels in the body.

Chapter 2: Histamine: Creation and Connection - Delves into the biochemistry of histamine, its production from the amino acid histidine, and its interactions with different receptors in the body.

Chapter 3: Histamine in the Immune Response - Examines the role of histamine in the immune system, focusing on mast cells and other immune cells that produce and release histamine.

Chapter 4: Unmasking Mast Cells - Provides an in-depth look at mast cells, their activation by various triggers, and the consequences of excessive mast cell activation.

Chapter 5: Histamine Balance: Genetics and More - Explores the genetic factors that influence histamine balance, including variations in the DAO, HNMT, and MTHFR genes.

Chapter 6: Gut Microbes Impact Histamine Levels - Investigates the role of the gut microbiome in regulating histamine levels and the potential impact of probiotics on histamine intolerance.

Chapter 7: Dietary Changes to Lower Histamine Levels - Offers practical advice on implementing a low-histamine diet and explores the connection between histamine and other dietary factors, such as FODMAPs and gluten.

Chapter 8: Natural Supplements for Reducing Histamine - Discusses various natural supplements that can help reduce histamine levels or stabilize mast cells, including quercetin, vitamin C, and DAO enzymes.

Chapter 9: Environmental and Lifestyle Factors - Examines the impact of environmental toxins, stress, and other lifestyle factors on histamine levels and mast cell activation.

Chapter 10: Over-the-Counter Medications - Provides an overview of over-the-counter medications that can help manage histamine-related symptoms, as well as those that may exacerbate histamine intolerance.

Chapter 11: Alcohol and Histamine - Explores the complex relationship between alcohol consumption and histamine levels, offering strategies for minimizing histamine reactions to alcohol.

Chapter 12: Histamine in the Brain - Investigates the role of histamine as a neurotransmitter and its involvement in various neurological conditions, such as migraines, depression, and anxiety.

Chapter 13: IBS, Acid Reflux, and Histamine - Examines the connection between histamine, irritable bowel syndrome (IBS), and acid reflux, providing insights into managing these conditions through histamine regulation.

Chapter 14: Sleep and Circadian Rhythm - Explores the relationship between histamine, sleep, and circadian rhythms, offering strategies for improving sleep quality by regulating histamine levels.

Chapter 15: Estrogen, Histamine, and Mast Cell Interaction - Delves into the complex interplay between estrogen, histamine, and mast cells, discussing the implications for women's health and hormone balance.

Chapter 16: Histamine, Asthma, and the Lungs - Examines the role of histamine in respiratory conditions, such as asthma, and explores the differences between allergic and non-allergic asthma.

Chapter 17: Bladder and Prostate Problems - Investigates the impact of histamine and mast cell activation on urological conditions, such as interstitial cystitis and prostate issues.

Part 1: Understanding Histamine

Chapter 1: Histamine Overload

Key takeaways:

- Symptoms of high histamine can include multiple body systems.
- Not everyone has the same symptoms when their histamine levels are high.
- Different terms can be used, such as histamine intolerance, high histamine symptoms, and mast cell activation syndrome.

Imagine feeling suddenly ill after a meal that others ate without issue, a recurring mystery that perplexes even your doctor. Or perhaps you have recurrent itching or problems with migraines. Welcome to the perplexing world of histamine-related health issues - where your experiences may defy a one-size-fits-all explanation. These seemingly unrelated symptoms, ranging from digestive issues to headaches, can all be tied to a common culprit: histamine intolerance. Understanding the various terms used to describe this condition is key to unraveling its complexities.

Whether it's called histamine intolerance, an imbalance where the body reacts to normal amounts of histamine in food, or mast cell activation syndrome, a condition where immune cells release too much histamine, the essence remains the same: an overabundance of histamine wreaking havoc in the body.

Let's unravel the mystery behind these labels and the wide range of symptoms they involve, shedding light on a condition that's as unique as the people it impacts.

Unravelling Histamine's Effects

Is it histamine intolerance, MCAS, pseudo-allergies, or high histamine symptoms? These terms all relate to high histamine levels due to different reasons. Let me explain what each of these means, and why I'm going to usually use high histamine levels as a general terminology.

While histamine intolerance is often used to describe symptoms triggered by ingesting histamine-rich foods, the reality is more nuanced. Let's take a closer look at the various terms used to describe histamine-related health issues and how they differ.

Experts define food intolerance as an abnormal response to a specific food at an amount that is normally tolerated. This is easy to understand for something like lactose intolerance, where a lack of an enzyme (lactase) makes it hard to digest the lactose found in dairy foods.

Histamine intolerance doesn't neatly fit the food intolerance definition. It isn't a reaction to just a specific food. Instead, it involves reactions to a component of many foods: histamine.

Histamine intolerance is a term that is applied mainly to reactions to histamine from food. Symptoms impact many systems in the body, including headaches, irritability, acid reflux, stomach pain, bloating, diarrhea, dizziness, sinus drainage, hives, itching, flushing, and insomnia.[1] People with histamine intolerance usually have several of the symptoms above, but they likely won't have all the symptoms.

There is an argument to be made that histamine intolerance isn't the right term. The problem can be more complex than symptoms caused by eating foods high in histamine! In fact, histamine from food is often just the tipping point, letting you know that there is an underlying problem with histamine imbalance.

While histamine intolerance primarily focuses on reactions to dietary histamine, mast cell activation syndrome (MCAS) takes histamine-related symptoms to a more systemic level. In MCAS, the body's mast cells release excessive amounts of histamine, leading to a wide array of symptoms. Regardless of the specific label used – histamine intolerance, MCAS, or simply high histamine levels – the common thread is an overabundance of histamine in the body. This excess histamine can manifest in various ways, affecting multiple body systems.

Throughout this book, I will include research from studies on high histamine levels, histamine intolerance, mast cell activation, and more. In general, I'll refer to them as high histamine symptoms to convey that for many people, the symptoms can be more than just a simple food intolerance.

---

[1] Schnedl et al., "Evaluation of Symptoms and Symptom Combinations in Histamine Intolerance."

Let's dive into the symptoms caused by high histamine levels.

High Histamine Symptoms:

Symptoms of high histamine vary and can affect multiple systems of the body. If you have problems with histamine intolerance or high histamine levels from any source, you may have some of these symptoms but not all.

Body systems impacted by high histamine levels include:[2]

Nervous system symptoms:

- Headaches and migraines
- Dizziness

Neurotransmitter symptoms:

- Insomnia, especially early morning waking
- Anxiety, irritability, or mood issues

Cardiovascular system symptoms:

- Tachycardia (rapid heart rate over 100 bpm)
- Arrhythmia
- Hypotonia of the heart muscle

Respiratory symptoms:

- Runny, drippy nose
- Sinus congestion
- Post-nasal drip, throat-clearing
- Shortness of breath
- Sneezing

Gastrointestinal system symptoms:

- Bloating and flatulence

---

[2] Hrubisko et al., "Histamine Intolerance—The More We Know the Less We Know. A Review."

- Feeling overly full after eating
- Diarrhea
- Abdominal pain
- Constipation
- Nausea and vomiting

Skin symptoms:

- Dermatographia
- Flushing
- Itching
- Hives
- Swelling
- Dermatitis

Again, people with histamine-related issues won't have all of those symptoms at once. Instead, they may be more prone to just a couple of areas of symptoms, such as sinus drainage and migraines, or heartburn and early morning insomnia.

Picture this: You're at your favorite pizza spot, indulging in a meat lover's feast. The rich flavors of sausage, pepperoni, and bacon linger as you sip your beer. But this meal comes with a hidden price for those with histamine intolerance! Pizza sauce, pepperoni, sausage, and bacon are all foods that are high in histamine, and the alcohol in the beer blocks the breakdown of histamine. Someone with histamine intolerance might have sinus drainage shortly after the meal, manifesting as throat clearing, or coughing on the way home from the restaurant. Perhaps heartburn starts a few hours later? Or just an uncomfortable feeling of over-fullness. Then there are the random, itchy little hives that appear out of nowhere by the next morning. Adding to the mix, a migraine or insomnia starts around 4 am.

Other people with histamine intolerance may find that they have more abdominal symptoms, such as stomach pain and nausea. Or they may find that high histamine foods alter their mood, making them more irritable or anxious. For some, histamine intolerance can be a few symptoms that come and go - like acid reflux or chronic sinus drainage. But other people may have much more severe allergy-like symptoms, such as chronic itching, hives, sinus infections, etc.[3]

Remember, everyone is unique in where their susceptibility to histamine-related symptoms lies. This is not a static condition that always results in the same symptoms.

Navigating Intolerance Diagnosis

You may think, I have all those histamine-related symptoms! Which doctor do I go to for a diagnosis? Is there a pill to fix it?

With such a wide range of potential symptoms, diagnosing histamine intolerance or MCAS can be a challenge. I know this can be overwhelming for many people, but a conversation with your trusted general physician is a good place to start. Even if they aren't familiar with histamine intolerance or histamine-related symptoms, they can help you rule out other diagnoses. Most of the high histamine symptoms overlap with other health issues, and your general physician can make sure you don't have something else going on.

An immunologist or allergy doctor may help with allergy testing, which can rule out or narrow down traditional IgE allergens.

A naturopathic physician or functional medicine doctor will be familiar with histamine intolerance and may be an excellent option for help, especially if you've ruled out other causes of your symptoms.

One reason many traditional physicians aren't eager to diagnose histamine intolerance is that there isn't a reliable diagnostic test and research studies show varied results by individuals.

---

[3] Hrubisko et al.

A review of histamine intolerance studies explains, "One may suggest that histamine-intolerant subjects reacted with different organs on different occasions. As a result, reproducibility of single symptoms alone may not be appropriate to diagnose histamine-intolerance whereas a global symptom score could be more appropriate."[4]

Histamine intolerance is frustrating to study and diagnose because of the variability in symptoms and the multiple systems that it can affect.

Acute Histamine Overdose:

What happens if you eat something with a ton of histamine and overdose on it? Well, you'll feel like you have food poisoning – scombroid poisoning, to be specific.

Consider scombroid poisoning as an extreme case of histamine overload. It's a severe reaction from seafood spoiled by high histamine levels, akin to an intense, rapid-onset gastrointestinal allergy. Symptoms include nausea, diarrhea, flushing, vertigo, itching, and faintness.

Fish and seafood can build up histamine levels quickly from bacterial contamination. Essentially, scombroid poisoning gives you a big dose of histamine along with other biogenic amines. The FDA has set a maximum allowable histamine level at 5 mg/ 100g of fish.[5]

Scombroid poisoning is an extreme example, showing the potent effects of histamine on the body and mirroring on a smaller scale what happens in histamine intolerance.

To illustrate the real-life impact of histamine-related health issues, let's explore the case of Claudia, a patient who benefitted from lowering histamine levels alongside other lifestyle changes.

---

[4] Komericki et al., "Histamine Intolerance."
[5] Al Bulushi et al., "Biogenic Amines in Fish."

Case Study: The Anxious Homemaker

By Dr. Ibby Omole

Claudia* is a pleasant 38-year-old anxious stay at home mom of two. She used to co-own a marketing agency but gave up her career 6 years ago when she had her first child. It was during this period that she suffered her first bout of depression. She was diagnosed with general anxiety disorder and postpartum depression. Her primary care physician put her on an antidepressant, and she felt somewhat better.

Over the years, she has been on and off different antidepressants. She had a second baby 3 years ago and went back on antidepressants due to feeling overwhelmed and extremely fatigued. She felt her entire body started to fall apart when she was diagnosed with mold toxicity 2 years prior.

She also had complaints of digestive issues such as gas, bloating, and several loose bowel movements a day. She was tested for SIBO which came back negative, but her *H. pylori* test was positive. She rated her stress at an 8/10 (10 is max) and her energy was a constant 3/10 (10 is high). Her most recent complaint was brain fog and loss of concentration. She did a lot of research and put herself on several supplements, but nothing seemed to be working.

Claudia's main goal was to just feel better again and have more energy to spend time with her husband and two children.

Genomic analysis using Genetic Lifehacks summary report showed that Claudia carried genetic variants for the breakdown of histamine in the digestive tract and systemically. In addition, she had SNPs (single nucleotide polymorphisms) for celiac disease, vitamin D deficiency, inflammatory bowel disease, IBS, leaky gut, and increased IgE response.

Of particular interest were genetic SNPs for HPA axis regulation, sleep, and mood.

Dietary Recommendations

- Low Histamine diet x 4 weeks to decrease the histamine load in the body

- Limit intake of fermented foods in the diet
- Limit the intake of histamine liberators such as citrus fruits
- Avoid preservatives and emulsifiers as they contribute to inflammation in the body
- Gluten free diet x 4 weeks to see if symptoms improve

Supplement Recommendation

- Vitamin D supplementation – stabilizes mast cells
- HistDAO – helps to downregulate histamine receptors in the body when taken regularly
- Combination product containing curcumin, resveratrol, quercetin, and black galingale – anti-inflammatory and anti-allergic. Prevents increase of mast cells in the digestive tract
- High quality multivitamin – helps to support the methylation pathway
- Mixed strain probiotic containing *Lactobacillus Rhamnosus*, *Bifidobacterium lactis* and *Saccharomyces boulardii*

Lifestyle Recommendations

- Cognitive Behavioral Therapy to help manage anxiety and feelings of overwhelm
- Yoga/Mindfulness meditation – 15 minutes in the morning and 15 minutes before bed
- Helps to regulate the nervous system and improve depression symptoms
- 20 minutes daily walk in nature to regulate the nervous system
- Blue light blocking glasses to help with difficulties falling asleep and help reset the circadian rhythm
- Bright light in the morning for at least 20 minutes to help reset the circadian rhythm

*Names and personal details are fictionalized in the case studies. These case studies are included to illustrate the different systems involved in histamine-related conditions. Please talk with your physician if you need advice or help with your situation.

Chapter 2: Histamine: Creation and Connection

Key takeaways:

- Histamine is a biogenic amine, formed from the amino acid histidine.
- Mast cells produce histamine at high levels; other cell types produce histamine at lower levels.
- There are four different histamine receptors that are activated by histamine, causing different actions to take place in the body.
- Two enzymes, DAO and HNMT, break down histamine and keep levels in balance.

Imagine histamine as a messenger in your body's communication network. It begins life as a simple amino acid, l-histidine, with vitamin B6 acting as the facilitator that transforms it into the powerful messenger known as histamine.

As we dive deeper, we'll explore how histamine interacts with its four types of receptors—H1, H2, H3, and H4—each playing a distinct part in translating histamine's message into physiological responses. The interaction of histamine with the four types of receptors is key to understanding histamine's diverse effects -- from allergy symptoms to sleep regulation; stomach acid production to immune system responses.

To fully grasp histamine's diverse effects on the body, it's essential to understand its chemical nature and how it interacts with various receptors. Let's start by exploring histamine's origin story as a biogenic amine.

Histamine's Origin Story

Histamine belongs to the biogenic amine family, a group of substances derived from amino acids — the building blocks of proteins. They contain an 'amine group,' a small molecule that is often included in chemical messengers in the body. The family of biogenic amines includes neurotransmitters - dopamine, serotonin, norepinephrine, and epinephrine - as well as polyamines such as cadaverine, putrescine, spermine, and spermidine.

Histidine is the amino acid that is used to make histamine, and it is one of the essential amino acids that we must get from foods. In addition to turning into histamine, muscle cells can use histidine to make carnosine and anserine, and histidine helps build the myelin sheath around nerves.

Foods high in histidine include most protein-rich foods, such as meat, fish, eggs, soy, and beans.[6]

From Amino Acid to Bioactive Messenger

How is Histamine Produced?

The conversion of histidine to histamine is facilitated by an enzyme called histidine decarboxylase, which is encoded by the HDC gene. You can think of the HDC enzyme as a specialized worker in your body's factory, tasked with transforming the raw material (histidine) into a versatile product (histamine).

Various cell types, including mast cells, basophils, neurons, gastrointestinal cells, and T cells, contain the HDC enzyme and use it to synthesize histamine. The conversion of histidine to histamine uses vitamin B6 as a cofactor.[7]

---

[6] Kessler and Raja, "Biochemistry, Histidine."
[7] Patel and Mohiuddin, "Biochemistry, Histamine."

Mast cells are like the emergency responders of your immune system, storing histamine in 'granules' ready to be dispatched at a moment's notice when an invader or an allergen is detected. In addition to their role in allergies and the immune response, mast cells are also responsible for most of the plasma histamine that circulates in the body.[8]

Macrophages, neutrophils, lymphocytes, keratinocytes, endothelial cells, and smooth muscle cells also contain the HDC enzyme, which can produce histamine when stimulated by inflammation. These cells cause a low-level, continual release of histamine, while mast cell degranulation causes quick, large amounts of histamine to be released.[9]

The cells in your stomach lining, called enterochromaffin-like cells, also produce histamine. When you eat (or are looking forward to eating), these cells release histamine. When histamine is in the stomach, it tells the body to release stomach acid by activating the H2 receptors on the cells that secrete gastric acid.

Other cell types that can produce histamine include basophils and lymphocytes, which are immune system cells, and neurons. Histamine can act as a neurotransmitter in the brain, produced by neurons to signal neighboring neurons.[10]

Adding an intriguing twist to the histamine story, the bacteria living in your gut also play a role in histamine production. Here are a couple of examples of how your microbiome interacts with histamine:

- Lactobacillus species and Klebsiella species produce histamine in the gut microbiome[11] [12]
- Alternatively, H. pylori infection in the stomach may inhibit histamine release.[13]

You'll find more details on how the gut microbiome affects histamine levels in Chapter 6.

---

8 Nakamura et al., "Regulation of Plasma Histamine Levels by the Mast Cell Clock and Its Modulation by Stress."

9 Hirasawa, "Expression of Histidine Decarboxylase and Its Roles in Inflammation."

10 Branco et al., "Role of Histamine in Modulating the Immune Response and Inflammation."

11 Pessione and Cirrincione, "Bioactive Molecules Released in Food by Lactic Acid Bacteria."

12 De Palma et al., "Histamine Production by the Gut Microbiota Induces Visceral Hyperalgesia through Histamine 4 Receptor Signaling in Mice."

13 Zaki et al., "H. Pylori Acutely Inhibits Gastric Secretion by Activating CGRP Sensory Neurons Coupled to Stimulation of Somatostatin and Inhibition of Histamine Secretion."

Decoding the Signal

Histamine exerts its effects by binding to four different types of receptors, which are like docking stations on cells throughout the body. These receptors, known as H1, H2, H3, and H4, are specialized G-coupled receptor proteins that function as switches. When histamine binds to these receptors, it triggers various cellular functions.

The variety of effects that histamine can cause depends on the type of cell and the type of histamine receptor. Each of the four histamine receptors plays a unique role in translating histamine's message into physiological responses.

Let's take a closer look at the function and effects of each receptor type to understand all of the different symptoms linked to high histamine levels.

H1 Receptor: The Allergy Alert

H1 receptor activation acts as a switch that activates the body's allergy response, resulting in symptoms like itching, redness, and mucous release.

Activation of H1 receptors can cause:[14]

- Itching
- Vasodilation (blood vessels dilate and become more permeable)
- Flushing
- Blood pressure drop
- Increased heart rate
- Bronchoconstriction, mucosal edema
- Mucous secretion

---

[14] Patel and Mohiuddin, "Biochemistry, Histamine."

The tissue in which histamine activates the receptor determines the effect. For example, H1 activation in the skin may cause itching, while activation in blood vessels may cause flushing or changes in blood pressure. In the lungs, activation of the H1 receptor causes bronchoconstriction, such as the narrowing of the airways that occurs during asthma attacks.

While the allergy-like symptoms are the most noticeable from H1 activation, the H1 receptors are also involved in:[15]

- Sleep/Wake cycles (being alert in the morning)
- Food intake (appetite and even anorexia)
- Emotions, aggression
- Thermal regulation
- Memory and learning
- Anaphylaxis

H2 Receptor: The Gastric Guardian

H2 receptors act like regulators in your stomach lining, telling your body when to pump out acid for digestion. They're also present in the heart and blood vessels, where they can influence your heartbeat and blood pressure.

Blocking the H2 receptor is a common way to stop heartburn caused by too much stomach acid. Commonly used H2 blocker medications include famotidine (brand name Pepcid in the U.S.) and cimetidine (brand name Tagamet).

Activation of H2 receptors can cause:

- Stomach acid secretion
- Vascular permeability
- Heart rate and blood pressure changes
- Headache
- Inhibition of some inflammatory responses[16]

---

[15] Lieberman, "The Basics of Histamine Biology."
[16] Hirasawa, "Expression of Histidine Decarboxylase and Its Roles in Inflammation."

H3 Receptor: The Neurological Gatekeeper

In the brain, the H3 receptor is present in histaminergic neurons. These neurons can regulate the release of neurotransmitters, including histamine, dopamine, serotonin, norepinephrine, and acetylcholine. The lungs and intestinal tract also contain H3 receptors.

Activation of H3 receptors can cause: [17]

- Modulation of brain histamine receptors
- Histamine release from mast cells
- Histamine release from neurons
- Inhibition of acetylcholine release in certain regions of the brain
- Bronchoconstriction, itching

Much of the research on the H3 receptor is relatively new, and there is probably more to learn about how the H3 receptor interacts with histamine and how H3 is blocked or activated by drugs or natural supplements that bind to it. However, the picture that is emerging is that the H3 receptor acts as a negative feedback regulator of histamine release in some tissues. While it is easy to get into the mindset of always wanting lower histamine levels, this may not be true in respect to histamine regulation in the brain by the H3 receptor. Balance is key.

H4 Receptor: The Immune Orchestrator

The H4 receptor is found on immune system cells such as monocytes, basophils, mast cells, basophils, T cells, and dendritic cells. Besides immune system cells, H4 receptors are also found on epithelial cells lining the gut.

Activation of the H4 receptor causes: [18]

- Activation of mast cells and eosinophils
- Differentiation of stem cells
- Itching (the chronic type found in atopic dermatitis)

---

[17] Branco et al., "Role of Histamine in Modulating the Immune Response and Inflammation."
[18] Schirmer and Neumann, "The Function of the Histamine H4 Receptor in Inflammatory and Inflammation-Associated Diseases of the Gut."

- Inflammation in the intestines in IBD, food allergy symptoms
- Release of DAO in the intestines with fat absorption

Histamine Receptors

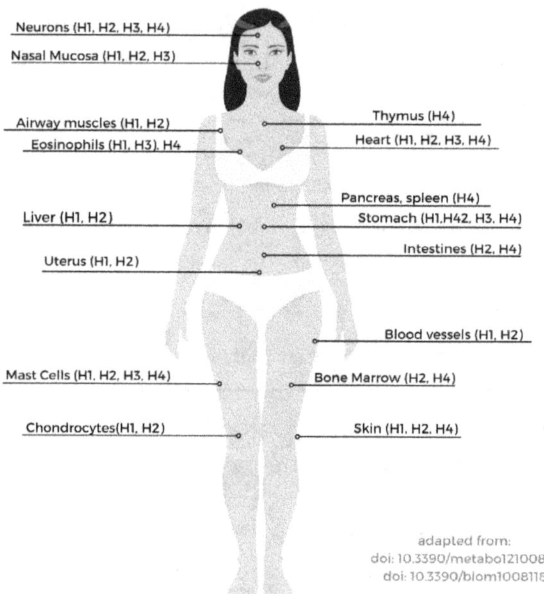

TRPV1 Receptor: The Pain and Itch Sensor

Expanding beyond histamine receptors, there's a sensory receptor called TRPV1 that acts as a versatile alarm, responding to both heat and irritation. Research shows that histamine can turn up the sensitivity of these alarms, leading to pain or itching. This TRPV1 activation is in conjunction with the H1 or H4 receptor on the nerve cell.[19]

---

[19] Wilzopolski et al., "TRPV1 and TRPA1 Channels Are Both Involved Downstream of Histamine-Induced Itch."

When TRPV1 is activated on peripheral nerves, like in your skin, it sends signals to your brain for pain or itching. In addition, research also shows that TRPV1 activation alongside histamine is involved in intestinal pain in IBS.

Understanding the diverse effects of histamine on the body through its interaction with different receptors underscores the importance of maintaining a delicate balance. In the next section, we'll explore how feedback loops and receptor sensitivity play a crucial role in regulating histamine levels.

Balancing the Histamine Scale

An often missed key concept in understanding histamine systems is the role of feedback loops.

Dealing with histamine-related symptoms can feel like being stuck on a rollercoaster, where histamine levels and receptor sensitivity constantly adjust to each other. The constant adjustments between histamine levels and receptor sensitivity create a dynamic feedback loop that lies at the heart of maintaining histamine balance.

On the one hand, you have the release of histamine from mast cells, the creation of histamine as a neurotransmitter, the release of histamine in the stomach, and the breakdown of histamine by DAO and HNMT. Together this regulates the amount of histamine in your system. But histamine doesn't act alone; the activated receptor is the key to histamine's actions. The other half of the picture here is the number of histamine receptors available on the surface of cells. When there are more histamine receptors available, they are more likely to be activated by circulating histamine.

Let me explain what I mean by feedback loops, receptors, and histamine levels with an example:

If you suffer from seasonal allergies, your nose might actually be ramping up its sensitivity by increasing the number of histamine receptors, amplifying your symptoms. Research shows that people with allergic rhinitis, which causes the runny nose and itchy, watery eyes in pollen allergies, have increased levels of H1 receptors in the cells that line the nose. Taking antihistamine medications that target the H1 receptor before allergy season prevents the upregulation of H1 receptors in the nose. This has been shown in studies to reduce allergy symptoms.[20]

Feedback loops and receptor sensitivity aren't limited to the H1 receptor and allergy symptoms. Histamine also plays many roles in the brain. A recent study of astrocytes, a type of glial cell, showed that increasing histamine levels caused a subsequent increase in H1, H2, and H3 receptors in these cells.[21]

Higher levels of histamine can upregulate the number of histamine receptors.

Let me restate that because this is important: If you have high levels of histamine from any source, your cells will respond by increasing the number of histamine receptors.[22] The upregulation of histamine receptors can be tissue-specific. After repeated exposure to something that increases histamine in your nose, you may develop more histamine receptors there. This would then increase your sensitivity to sinus drainage.

For example, repeated exposure to pollen, dust mites, or an environmental allergen could increase histamine release in the nose. Similarly, exposure to a chemical irritant, such as a strong solvent, could do the same. Animal studies show that repeated exposure to chemicals, such as the solvent toluene-2,4-diisocyanate (TDI), leads to an upregulation of H1 receptors in the nose.[23]

---

[20] Mizuguchi et al., "Signaling Pathway of Histamine H1 Receptor-Mediated Histamine H1 Receptor Gene Upregulation Induced by Histamine in U-373 MG Cells."

[21] Xu et al., "Histamine Upregulates the Expression of Histamine Receptors and Increases the Neuroprotective Effect of Astrocytes."

[22] Mizuguchi et al., "Signaling Pathway of Histamine H1 Receptor-Mediated Histamine H1 Receptor Gene Upregulation Induced by Histamine in U-373 MG Cells."

[23] Shahriar et al., "Suplatast Tosilate Inhibits Histamine Signaling by Direct and Indirect Down-Regulation of Histamine H1 Receptor Gene Expression through Suppression of Histidine Decarboxylase and IL-4 Gene Transcriptions1."

Blocking the histamine receptor, such as the H1 receptor, with an over-the-counter antihistamine, can also downregulate the receptor. For example, pretreatment with a nasal antihistamine before exposure to pollen reduces the allergic symptoms.[24]

However, blocking the H1 receptor doesn't reduce the total amount of histamine produced in the allergic reaction, so for someone who doesn't break down histamine well, this may lead to histamine symptoms elsewhere in the body. While reducing histamine levels may help to keep receptors from being upregulated, the converse isn't true. Importantly, research also shows that DAO enzyme production is not downregulated on a low histamine diet.[25]

When histamine is no longer needed as a signaling molecule, how do we break down and eliminate it? Let's explore the two key enzymes responsible for maintaining histamine balance: DAO and HNMT.

Clearing Histamine from the Body:

To maintain optimal histamine levels, the body primarily uses two enzymes: diamine oxidase (DAO) and histamine N-methyltransferase (HNMT). These two enzymes help to keep histamine at the right level in the various tissues of the body.[26]

1. **Diamine oxidase (DAO) enzyme:** Histamine from food or bacteria in your intestines is broken down or metabolized by the enzyme DAO (diamine oxidase). The DAO enzyme is produced in the villi that line the small intestine and is released to metabolize histamine.
2. **Histamine methyltransferase (HNMT) enzyme:** The HNMT enzyme works throughout the body, including in the brain, to deactivate and break down histamine produced by your cells.

24 Fukui et al., "Histamine H1 Receptor Gene Expression and Drug Action of Antihistamines."
25 Son et al., "A Histamine-Free Diet Is Helpful for Treatment of Adult Patients with Chronic Spontaneous Urticaria."
26 Yoshikawa, Nakamura, and Yanai, "Histamine N-Methyltransferase in the Brain," February 10, 2019.

1. Diamine oxidase (DAO) enzyme:

The blueprint for creating the DAO enzyme, which breaks down histamine from your food, is the AOC1 gene. DAO is primarily produced in the intestines as a response to histamine from food and intestinal bacteria. Foods high in histamine include aged cheeses, aged meats, fermented foods, and more. (More details on high histamine foods are in Chapter 7.)

Histamine-producing bacteria in the gut, including those found in some probiotics or fermented foods, can also increase histamine levels in the body. Researchers have found that people with histamine intolerance have altered gut microbiome composition and elevated levels of zonulin, which regulates tight junctions in the gut (leaky gut).[27] Another recent study of histamine intolerance patients found they had "a significantly higher abundance of histamine-secreting bacteria".[28]

The body also used the DAO enzyme to break down other biogenic amines, including tyramine, putrescine, cadaverine, spermidine, and spermine. High levels of other biogenic amines can reduce DAO's ability to break down histamine.[29]

DAO degrades histamine to imidazole acetaldehyde. This is then rapidly oxidized to imidazole acetic acid.

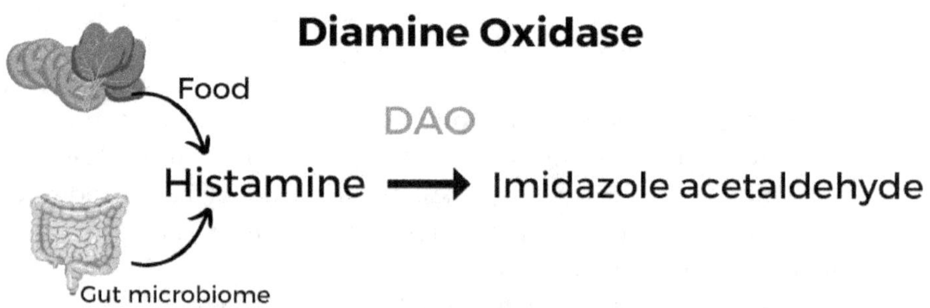

---

[27] "Microbial Patterns in Patients with Histamine Intolerance."
[28] Sánchez-Pérez et al., "Intestinal Dysbiosis in Patients with Histamine Intolerance."
[29] Sánchez-Pérez et al., "The Rate of Histamine Degradation by Diamine Oxidase Is Compromised by Other Biogenic Amines," May 25, 2022.

While DAO primarily targets histamine from food and intestinal bacteria, HNMT works throughout the body to deactivate and break down histamine produced by your cells. Let's take a closer look at how HNMT contributes to histamine balance.

2. HNMT enzyme:

The HNMT enzyme breaks down histamine throughout the body including in the brain where histamine levels are tightly controlled as a neurotransmitter.

The HNMT enzyme is also expressed in the liver, kidney, skin, spleen, colon, prostate, ovary, and lung. Genetically reduced HNMT is also associated with atopic dermatitis or eczema and an increased risk of asthma. While DAO can also circulate in the periphery, HNMT is the only enzyme that breaks down the neurotransmitter histamine in the central nervous system.[30]

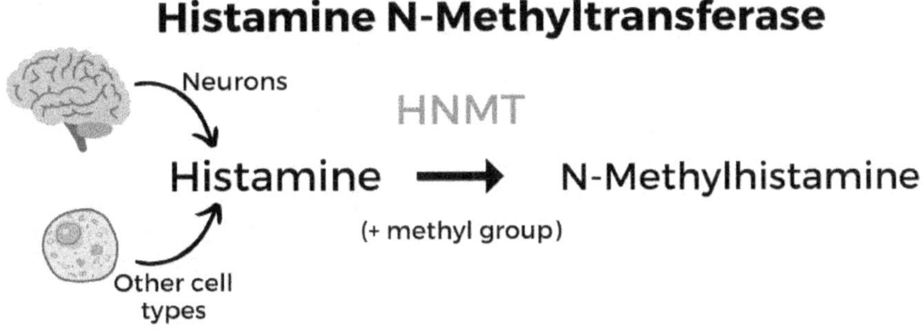

When histamine is degraded by the HNMT enzyme, it forms N-methylhistamine with the addition of a methyl group. The availability of methyl groups is important here, and we will come back to this in Chapter 5 with genetic variants that impact the availability of methyl groups.

---

[30] Maintz and Novak, "Histamine and Histamine Intolerance2."

The N-methylhistamine is further broken down by the MAO-B enzyme to form N-methylimidazole acetaldehyde. Research shows that the MAO-B enzyme doesn't break down histamine under normal conditions, but when HNMT is inhibited, MAO-B can step in and help metabolize histamine in the brain.[31]

Genetic variants that alter HNMT levels show us the many impacts of histamine throughout the brain. For example, altered HNMT levels in the brain are associated with an increased risk of neurodegenerative diseases, such as Parkinson's disease. Genetically decreased HNMT levels can increase histamine levels. Studies link HNMT variants to an increased risk of migraines and ADHD. Conversely, low levels of HNMT may be protective against neurodegenerative diseases in aging.

Genes make everyone unique in their response to histamine. You'll find more details on the genetic variants in Chapter 5.

---

[31] Maršavelski et al., "Why Monoamine Oxidase B Preferably Metabolizes N-Methylhistamine over Histamine."

Chapter 3: Histamine in the Immune Response

Key takeaways:

- Histamine is an essential part of the innate immune response.
- Mast cells release large amounts of histamine as part of their response to a pathogen or allergen.
- Other immune cells, such as macrophages and neutrophils, can also synthesize and release histamine.

Before we dive deeper into all the ways excess histamine causes trouble, let's first look at its critical role in the body's immune response. Histamine is a vital player in your body's first line of defense – the innate immune system. While we often focus on the negative aspects of too much histamine, it is important to also understand why we need the right amount of histamine available at a moment's notice.

As a crucial player in the body's first line of defense, histamine is involved in various aspects of the immune response. Let's explore how histamine interacts with different immune system components to protect the body from pathogens and foreign substances.

Mast cells are like the immune system's first responders, always ready to release histamine at the first sign of trouble. When a pathogen, such as a virus, or an allergen activates mast cells, they immediately release histamine. A common example is a mosquito bite—the redness, swelling, and itching you experience are all due to mast cells unleashing histamine in response to the insect's saliva. Histamine then acts like a signal flare, causing nearby blood vessels to widen (a process known as vasodilation) and become 'leakier', making it easier for white blood cells to rush to the scene. The increased vascular permeability allows for the passaging of white blood cells and other immune system factors to the site of inflammation.

Histamine plays both an inflammatory and anti-inflammatory role in the immune response. By binding to different receptors, histamine can either promote or suppress inflammation, depending on the context. Both roles are important for an effective innate immune response against pathogens and foreign substances.[32]

Mast Cells: The Immune System's First Responders

Much like emergency teams that rush to the scene of a crisis, mast cells spring into action at the first sign of invasion or injury. While I'll go into more detail about mast cells in Chapter 4, I wanted to briefly explain that mast cells are part of our body's innate defense against all types of pathogens, known and unknown.

Mast cells are stationed in high-risk areas of your body – skin, nose, lungs, and gut – ready to sound the alarm and mount a defense at a moment's notice. They can react almost instantly to viruses, bacteria, parasites, toxins, damaged cells, and foreign substances (including allergens that the body mistakes for foreign). The release of histamine triggers a cascade of events, from increased vascular permeability to signaling for an inflammatory cascade. All of this brings an immediate immune response to the area of mast cell activation - essential for fighting a broad class of pathogens.

A recently discovered receptor, the MRGPRX2 receptor, has been found to trigger mast cells' defense against a variety of threats, including bee venom and certain medications.

While mast cells are the primary source of histamine in the immune response, other immune cells, such as basophils and natural killer cells, can also contribute to histamine production. Let's take a closer look at some specific examples of non-mast cell immune system reactions involving histamine.

---

[32] Branco et al., "Role of Histamine in Modulating the Immune Response and Inflammation."

Beyond Mast Cells: Other Histamine Sources

In addition to mast cells, other immune players like basophils and natural killer cells also produce histamine. Skin cells can also produce histamine without involving mast cells, and this often results in more prolonged, chronic types of reactions, such as persistent itching. This type of reaction is still an important part of the immune response to toxins or chemicals that could be harmful to the body.

Here are a couple of examples of non-mast cell immune system reactions:

Dermatitis:
Animal studies show that adding an irritant or surfactant to the skin, such as sodium laureth sulfate, for an extended period can cause chronic itching. This type of skin reaction was found to be due to histamine released directly from skin cells, including keratinocytes, and not from mast cells. Other studies show that dust mites, TNF-alpha, and even certain bacteria can stimulate histamine release from skin cells.[33]

Metal-induced inflammation:
Researchers have found that nickel allergy can be caused by nickel exposure to the skin. Animal research points to nickel allergy being independent of mast cells. Constant exposure to nickel can cause HDC enzyme upregulation and histamine production in skin cells along with other inflammatory cytokines.[34]

Histamine's Strategic Immune Tactics

Histamine receptors, including H1 and H2 receptors, are found on the surface of many types of immune system cells. Activation of these receptors plays a role in the differentiation of T cells, B cells, monocytes, and dendritic cells during allergic inflammation.

---

[33] Hirasawa, "Expression of Histidine Decarboxylase and Its Roles in Inflammation."
[34] Kishimoto et al., "Induced Histamine Regulates Ni Elution from an Implanted Ni Wire in Mice by Downregulating Neutrophil Migration."

When Th1 cells are activated by histamine binding to the H1 receptor, it results in the synthesis and release of interferon-gamma, an inflammatory cytokine. This ramps up the allergic inflammatory response. However, the binding of histamine to the H2 receptors on Th2 cells causes a suppression in cell function.[35]

Histamine's role in modulating immune response, including the balance of Th1 and Th2 cells, is important in keeping the inflammatory response balanced -- strong enough to fight off pathogens but not overactive.

---

[35] Patel and Mohiuddin, "Biochemistry, Histamine."

Case Study: The Itchy Social Worker

Cindy is a 33-year-old female with a long history of eczema and asthma. She reported that her face and neck always get very itchy, especially after a very hot shower. The eczema is more pronounced on her face, behind the knees and in front of the elbows. She is very sensitive to skin care products including natural oils. She has environmental allergies to grass, pollen, cats, dogs, and horses.

Cindy mentioned that her stress has been very high lately due to an increased workload and some workplace drama. She has noticed that as she gets older, her eczema seems to get worse. Lately she has been getting migraines and insomnia particularly around ovulation time. She has also noticed an increase in gas, bloating, abdominal cramps, and loose stools closer to the beginning of her menstrual cycle.

Cindy finds her job as a social worker very stressful and has noticed that whenever she is stressed her digestive and menstrual issues get worse.

Six months prior to the appointment, she started breaking out in hives whenever she was exposed to extreme hot or cold temperatures. This is causing significant amounts of distress as she is unable to exercise or go outdoors without having a reaction. She also started experiencing some dizziness in addition to heaviness in her chest. Lastly her hands and feet are constantly cold, and she was told she has hypothyroidism.

She cut out caffeine, alcohol, nightshades, gluten, and dairy from her diet. She cut out gluten because she noticed an increase in eczema flare up whenever she ate gluten.

Genomic analysis showed that she did not have variants for celiac disease or wheat sensitivity/intolerance. However, she did have genetic variants that affected the clearance of histamine from the digestive tract and systemically. She was also more likely to have leaky gut and inflammatory bowel disease. Additionally, she had variants for lactose intolerance and sensitivity to nightshades and pesticides. Lastly, she didn't detoxify estrogen well from her system.

Supplement Recommendations

- Quercetin + Vitamin C combination product
- DIM + Sulforaphane + Calcium D glucarate product
  - Helps support liver detoxification to lower estrogen levels in the body
  - Estrogen increases the release of histamine from mast cells
- Vitamin D - helps stabilize mast cells
- HistDAO - taken daily to help increase the breakdown on histamine in the digestive tract
- High quality multivitamin - helps to support the methylation pathway and clearance of histamine from the bloodstream
- Combination product with Holy Basil, GABA and L-theanine to help decrease cortisol in the body and lower anxiety
- Multi-strain *Lactobacillus*, *Bifidobacterium*, and *Saccharomyces boulardii* probiotic to help decrease inflammation in the digestive tract

Dietary Recommendations

- Whole foods anti-inflammatory diet that is high in fruits and vegetables with lean grass-fed meats
  - Remove processed foods from the diet
  - Eliminate foods in the nightshade family (peppers, tomatoes, potatoes, and eggplant) for 3 months
  - Eliminate lactose containing foods in the diet
  - Eat a mostly organic diet
  - Use dirty dozen, clean fifteen guide to help choose produce that has a lower pesticide residue
  - Add more nuts and seeds that are high in Omega 3 fatty acids
  - Include foods that are in the cruciferous family (arugula, cabbage, Brussels sprouts, broccoli, kale) for their detoxifying properties

- No alcoholic beverages for 3 months

While her Genetic Lifehacks Summary report did not show any variants for Celiac disease or wheat sensitivity, it is possible that the reaction she noticed with gluten is from pesticides that were sprayed on the crop. Research has shown that certain pesticides can lead to the release of histamine within the body.[36]

Lifestyle Recommendations

- Mindfulness Meditation for 15 mins in the morning and 15 minutes at night
  - Choose personal care products that do not contain xenoestrogens
  - Recommended using the EWG website or Yuka app to source less toxic personal care products
- Focus on gentle body movements such as stretching, yoga, or pilates for 2 months

---

[36] Sato et al., "Augmentation of Allergic Reactions by Several Pesticides."

Chapter 4: Unmasking Mast Cells

Key takeaways:

- Mast cells are immune cells that can quickly react to perceived invaders by releasing histamine, tryptase, and cytokines.
- IgE antibodies can trigger the activation of mast cells during allergic reactions.
- Environmental chemicals, viruses, bacteria, and physical stimulation can also activate mast cells.
- Too many mast cells or their easy activation can cause an excess of histamine in the body.

Let's go more in-depth on the topic of mast cells and explore how they work, where they come from, and what role they play in the body. This chapter will help you understand how mast cell activation leads to histamine release and discuss the many ways in which mast cells can be activated.

Mast Cells: Diving Deep

To fully appreciate the impact of mast cells on histamine levels and the body's overall function, it's essential to understand their unique characteristics and the mechanisms behind their activation.

Mast cells are a type of immune cell that creates, stores, and releases histamine, along with other substances. Most tissues in the body contain mast cells, but they are particularly abundant in areas of the body exposed to the outside world, such as the skin, nose, eyes, intestinal tract, and even blood vessels.

Think of mast cells as special agents in the army of your white blood cells. They are triggered to release large amounts of histamine and other mediators in the following circumstances:

- When presented with an allergen (IgE activation). This is the typical allergic mechanism.
- If activated by protozoa, helminth (worms)[37], or bacterial particles (lipopolysaccharides)
- When amplified by platelet-activating factor, a mediator of platelet aggregation and anaphylaxis.[38]

Picture a mast cell as a balloon filled with countless tiny beads, or granules. Each of these granules is a miniature storage unit, packed with an array of substances ready to be released when the body sends the signal. Mast cells are relatively large, housing between 50 and 200 granules that contain histamine, heparin, tryptase, inflammatory cytokines, and chondroitin sulfate—a potent cocktail of compounds that can have a profound impact on the body. When activated, they can release relatively large amounts of these mediators almost instantaneously. This is beneficial in combating pathogens, but it can also be responsible for allergic reactions and anaphylaxis.[39]

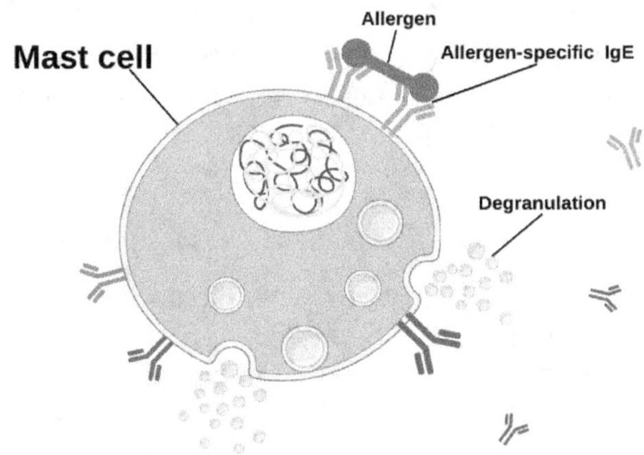

---

[37] Webb and Tait Wojno, "The Role of Rare Innate Immune Cells in Type 2 Immune Activation against Parasitic Helminths."
[38] Munoz-Cano et al., "Effects of Rupatadine on Platelet- Activating Factor-Induced Human Mast Cell Degranulation Compared With Desloratadine and Levocetirizine (The MASPAF Study)."
[39] Krystel-Whittemore, Dileepan, and Wood, "Mast Cell."

Mast Cell Activation Syndrome OR Histamine Intolerance?

At the beginning of this book, I mentioned that there are multiple terms applied to histamine-related symptoms. Some will refer to histamine intolerance while others may talk nebulously about mast cell activation syndrome. While mast cells are usually involved in high histamine levels, let's dive into more formal definitions of mast cell-related diseases.

Mast cell activation syndrome (MCAS) is caused by the systemic overactivation of mast cells. This means that MCAS happens when mast cells in your body react too strongly and too often.

Diagnostic symptoms include flushing, blood pressure dropping, itching, runny nose, headache, diarrhea, hives, swelling, or wheezing. For an MCAS diagnosis, at least two organ systems need to be involved (e.g., lungs, skin, gastrointestinal) along with recurring episodes with no other cause.[40]

Other terms, such as Mast Cell Activation Disorder (MCAD) and Mast Cell Disorder (MCD), are also used to describe similar symptoms. On the other hand, mastocytosis is a separate condition where a gain-of-function genetic mutation causes increased production of mast cells in tissues.

How does histamine intolerance differ from mast cell activation syndrome?

A few researchers categorize histamine intolerance as a subset of mast cell activation syndrome (MCAS). However, most consider it a separate diagnosis that mainly applies to symptoms triggered by high histamine foods. Those defining histamine intolerance as more strictly food-related describe it primarily as a lack of production of DAO enzyme. However you define it, the release of histamine from mast cells plays a role in high histamine levels for many people. Now, let's explore the various triggers that can cause mast cells to release their contents, leading to a surge in histamine levels.

---

[40] Giannetti et al., "Mast Cell Activation Disorders."

Triggering Mast Cell Degranulation:

Mast cells contain granules filled with ready-to-release histamine, tryptase, and inflammatory cytokines. They are 'pre-formed', meaning that they are ready to roll when triggered. This makes mast cells a first line of defense, able to be instantly released in response to a pathogen or foreign substance.

Mast cell triggers include:

- **Traditional Allergens**: Common allergens, like pollen, can set mast cells into action.
- **Pathogens**: Viruses and bacteria are detected and tackled by mast cells.
- **Chemical Exposure**: Everyday chemicals may inadvertently trigger a mast cell response.
- **Physical Stimulation**: Surprisingly, even vibrations can prompt mast cells to release their contents.

Let's go into each of these in more detail.

Allergies and mast cells:

In classical allergic reactions, the immune system produces immunoglobulin E (IgE) antibodies in response to an allergen, such as pollen or dust mites. These IgE antibodies then seek out and bind to specific receptors on the surface of mast cells. Like a key fitting into a lock, the interaction between the IgE antibody and its receptor triggers the activation of the mast cell, leading to the release of histamine and other inflammatory mediators

Mast cells are the body's lookouts stationed in high-risk areas like the skin and the lining of the lungs and gut, where threats from the outside world are most likely to strike. Activation of mast cells in these areas produces what we think of as allergic reaction symptoms, such as itchy skin, rash, airway hypersensitivity, anaphylaxis, and diarrhea.

If you have allergies, you may find that exposure to the allergen also aggravates your histamine intolerance symptoms. For example, during the spring pollen season, you may find that you react more easily to histamine-rich foods. This may be due to an increase in overall histamine levels in the body, triggered by allergens that activate mast cells.[41]

While allergens are well-known triggers of mast cell activation, it's important to recognize that viruses and bacteria can also provoke a similar response. In the next section, we'll examine how these pathogens interact with mast cells and contribute to histamine release.

Viruses and bacteria that activate mast cells:

Mast cells spring into action against viruses, bacteria, and fungi. This rapid response is a key part of how your body fights off these invaders.[42] However, for someone with chronically high histamine, an excessive mast cell response could exacerbate the symptoms of a mild viral infection. In addition, an ongoing low-level infection could contribute to the release of histamine by mast cells.

Here are some examples of how mast cells interact with viruses:

- Lyme disease, specifically *Borrelia burgdorferi* spirochetes, causes mast cells to release histamine.[43]
- Influenza A, the virus that causes the flu, increases histamine release and can trigger mast cell degranulation.[44]
- *H. pylori* is a common viral infection of the stomach that can cause ulcers. Recent studies show that *H. pylori* can activate mast cells and cause chronic itching and hives.[45]
- A substance called lipopolysaccharide, found on some bacteria, can make mast cells react even more. In people with asthma or

---

41 Winther et al., "Basophil Histamine Release, IgE, Eosinophil Counts, ECP, and EPX Are Related to the Severity of Symptoms in Seasonal Allergic Rhinitis."
42 Piliponsky, Acharya, and Shubin, "Mast Cells in Viral, Bacterial, and Fungal Infection Immunity."
43 Talkington and Nickell, "Borrelia Burgdorferi Spirochetes Induce Mast Cell Activation and Cytokine Release."
44 Graham, Temple, and Obar, "Mast Cells and Influenza a Virus."
45 Zaki et al., "H. Pylori Acutely Inhibits Gastric Secretion by Activating CGRP Sensory Neurons Coupled to Stimulation of Somatostatin and Inhibition of Histamine Secretion."

other mast cell-related diseases, exposure to lipopolysaccharide exacerbates symptoms.[46]

Environmental chemicals and physical stimulation

Everyday items around us can also trigger mast cell degranulation. This includes certain chemicals in plastics and metals. Research shows that PFAS (polyfluorinated substances, BPA (in plastics), sodium fluoride, and heavy metals, along with mold and mycotoxins, are also mast cell triggers for many people.

Movement, vibration, and physical stimulation can cause histamine release. I'll cover this further in chapter 9, but here is a brief overview:

Acupuncture:
When you receive acupuncture, it's not just the needles at work. Histamine released from mast cells at an acupuncture point plays a role in how acupuncture works. Acupuncture points in traditional Chinese medicine are places where mast cells are abundant. The needles or pressure on the acupuncture point causes histamine to be released from the mast cell, which in turn, activates the receptor of the nerve cells in the area.[47]

Exercise:
Histamine is released during exercise, particularly aerobic exercise. Mast cells release histamine to dilate the blood vessels surrounding skeletal muscle. This causes vasodilation, bringing more oxygen to the muscles and subsequently lowering blood pressure after exercise.[48]

[46] Kumari, Dash, and Singh, "Lipopolysaccharide (LPS) Exposure Differently Affects Allergic Asthma Exacerbations and Its Amelioration by Intranasal Curcumin in Mice."
[47] Yin et al., "A Mathematical Model of Histamine-Mediated Neural Activation during Acupuncture."
[48] Romero et al., "Mast Cell Degranulation and de Novo Histamine Formation Contribute to Sustained Postexercise Vasodilation in Humans."

Hives (urticaria) due to vibration:
Some people may experience vibratory urticaria due to repeated exposure to vibrations, such as when using hand tools. Researchers have found that a genetic variant in the ADGRE2 gene can cause vibratory urticaria. This gene encodes an epidermal growth factor that is crucial in skin cell signaling. The genetic variant alters the ADGRE2 gene, making it more susceptible to shear stress from vibration. The change to the ADGRE2 gene causes increased sensitivity in mast cells to vibration-induced degranulation, which results in a systemic increase in histamine levels.[49]

MRGPRX2 Receptor Activation

Some people seem to react more easily to everything from medications to bacteria that are commonly found on the skin. Often called hypersensitivity reactions, these non-allergy activations of mast cells can leave you scratching your head, wondering why you react to everything.

Recent advancements in mast cell research have uncovered a novel receptor called MRGPRX2, which adds another layer of complexity to the activation of these cells. Unlike the classic IgE-mediated pathway, MRGPRX2 represents a non-IgE route for mast cell activation. When triggered, this receptor initiates a cascade of events that culminates in mast cell degranulation and the consequent release of histamine and other inflammatory compounds.

Activation of MRGPRX2:

MRGPRX2 activation is implicated in various chronic conditions such as rosacea, asthma, atopic dermatitis, rheumatoid arthritis, and ulcerative colitis. The MRGPRX2 receptor can be activated by a variety of substances, including:

- Antimicrobial peptides
- Bacterial quorum-sensing molecules
- Protein fragments
- Neuropeptides like substance P
- Venom peptides (bee venom)

---

[49] Boyden et al., "Vibratory Urticaria Associated with a Missense Variant in ADGRE2."

- Certain medications

For example, research shows that a skin infection with commonly found dermal bacteria is detected by the MRGPRX2 receptor. The MRGPRX2 is thought to play a role in rosacea, as well. While rosacea involves more than just mast cell activation, studies of rosacea patients show that they have higher numbers and more activated mast cells than normal.[50]

Medication-Induced MRGPRX2 Activation

Several drugs can induce hypersensitivity reactions through MRGPRX2 activation, including:[51]

- Fluoroquinolone antibiotics
- Opiates
- Neuromuscular blocking agents used in anesthesia
- Iodinated contrast media used in medical imaging

These reactions are often dose-dependent and more likely to occur with intravenous administration.

The recent discovery of the MRGPRX2 receptor helps to explain the activation of mast cells in ways that were traditionally not understood. It also is a good reminder that much of the research on histamine-related symptoms and mast cells is constantly evolving, with new research coming out all the time. This story is still being written.

---

[50] Roy et al., "Multifaceted MRGPRX2."
[51] Ayudhya and Ali, "MRGPRX2 and Its Role in Non-IgE-Mediated Drug Hypersensitivity."

Chapter 5: Histamine Balance: Genetics and More

Key takeaways:

- Histamine levels need to be balanced between intake, production, and elimination.
- Imbalance can be caused by genetic variants, usually in combination with other factors.
- DAO and HNMT enzymes are needed in the right amount to break down histamine for elimination.
- Excess production of histamine can tip the scales.

To maintain optimal histamine levels, the body relies on two crucial enzymes: diamine oxidase (DAO) and histamine N-methyltransferase (HNMT). Let's explore how genetic variations in the genes encoding these enzymes can influence an individual's susceptibility to histamine imbalance.

High histamine symptoms occur when the histamine system is imbalanced. This can be caused by two main factors:

1. Not enough of the enzymes needed to break down histamine (DAO and HNMT enzymes)
   - and/or -
2. Too much histamine is being produced (HDC genetic variants, gut microbiome, high histamine foods, mast cells degranulating too easily, chronic exposure to allergens).

Imagine a scale with histamine production on one side and histamine degradation on the other — it all needs to balance out. Figuring out which side of the scale you need to work on can help you prioritize where to focus first.

To break down histamine, the body requires the DAO and HNMT enzymes. Not producing enough of the enzymes, due to genetics, can be one factor in histamine-related symptoms. Additionally, medications that you take may decrease your ability to produce the enzymes.

The other side of the equation is that some people genetically are geared toward creating more histamine due to variants in the HDC gene.

Just as our genes determine our hair color or height, they also shape our body's response to histamine, sometimes making us more sensitive to it. For most people, histamine issues are neither solely genetic nor solely due to environmental or gut microbiome factors. Instead, it is the combination that leads someone to be susceptible to histamine imbalance.

Diamine Oxidase (DAO) Enzyme

Diamine oxidase is encoded by the AOC1 gene. It is mainly produced in the cells lining the intestines to directly counteract histamine from foods and histamine created by intestinal bacteria. The DAO enzyme degrades histamine into imidazole acetaldehyde, which is then quickly oxidized into imidazole acetic acid for excretion.

In addition to being produced in the mucous membrane lining the intestines, DAO is also produced in the kidneys and in the placenta during pregnancy. Essentially, DAO is abundant in the intestines to break histamine down before it is absorbed and transported throughout the body. Keep in mind that histamine in the gut is both from histamine-containing foods and from gut bacteria that produce histamine.

A deficiency of the DAO enzyme can be due to several factors:[52]

- Genetic variants that cause lower DAO production.
- Drugs that cause impaired DAO activity
- Gastrointestinal disorders that damage the intestines such as celiac, IBS, or IBD
- Overproduction of other biogenic amines

Let's get into the genetic reasons for decreased DAO production here, and then we will touch on the other causes of reduced DAO.

---

[52] Neree et al., "Vegetal Diamine Oxidase Alleviates Histamine-Induced Contraction of Colonic Muscles."

AOC1 gene and a genetic reduction of DAO:

Imagine your body's ability to break down histamine as a highway. Genetic variants are like construction zones on this highway - they can slow down the traffic flow, which in this case is the breakdown of histamine.

Genetic inheritance plays a significant role in determining an individual's DAO enzyme production. Just as genetic variants can influence physical traits like eye or hair color, variations in the AOC1 gene, which provides the blueprint for the diamine oxidase enzyme, can impact the body's ability to produce DAO. Research shows that certain variants in the AOC1 gene affect histamine levels along with the risk of histamine-related conditions.

Genetic variants are tracked by researchers through an identification system consisting of "rs" plus a unique number. This gives researchers a common way to identify and talk about a change in a gene. For example, rs10156191 is a genetic variant that causes reduced production of DAO.[53] Similarly, the rs2052129 variant in the AOC1 gene is also associated with a reduced production of DAO. Research links both variants to an increased risk of migraines due to excess histamine.[54]

Not everyone with an AOC1 genetic variant will have histamine intolerance, and not everyone with histamine intolerance has these genetic variants. Instead, the AOC1 genetic variants increase the risk of histamine intolerance but aren't the sole cause. For most, it is a combination of a genetic decrease in DAO combined with other factors, such as gut microbiome changes or increased production of histamine by mast cells.

If you have genetic data from 23andMe, AncestryDNA, or a similar service, you can check your raw data to see if you have AOC1 genetic variants.

---

[53] Maintz et al., "Association of Single Nucleotide Polymorphisms in the Diamine Oxidase Gene with Diamine Oxidase Serum Activities."
[54] García-Martín et al., "Diamine Oxidase Rs10156191 and Rs2052129 Variants Are Associated with the Risk for Migraine."

Check your genetic data for **rs10156191**:

- C/C: typical genotype
- C/T: reduced production of the DAO enzyme[55]
- T/T: reduced production of the DAO enzyme[56]

Check your genetic data for **rs2052129**:

- G/G: typical (most common genotype)
- G/T: reduced production of DAO, increased risk of migraines due to histamine[57]
- T/T: reduced production of DAO[58], increased risk of migraines due to histamine

Check your genetic data for **rs1049742**:

- C/C: typical
- C/T: reduced production of DAO
- T/T: reduced production of DAO[59]

Check your genetic data for **rs1049793**:

- C/C: typical, high
- C/G: reduced production of DAO (35% reduction)
- G/G: reduced production of DAO (50% reduction)[60]

---

[55] García-Martín et al.

[56] García-Martín et al.

[57] García-Martín et al.

[58] Maintz et al., "Association of Single Nucleotide Polymorphisms in the Diamine Oxidase Gene with Diamine Oxidase Serum Activities."

[59] García-Martín et al., "Diamine Oxidase Rs10156191 and Rs2052129 Variants Are Associated with the Risk for Migraine."

[60] Ayuso et al., "Genetic Variability of Human Diamine Oxidase."

Check your genetic data for **rs2071514**:

- A/A: possibly higher DAO[61]
- A/G: possibly higher DAO
- G/G: typical

While genetic factors can influence DAO production, it's important to recognize that certain medications can also hinder the enzyme's function. In the next two sections, we'll look at how specific drugs can interfere with DAO activity and how other biogenic amines can exacerbate histamine imbalance.

Drugs that impair DAO production

Certain drugs can put a damper on DAO (diamine oxidase), much like a wrench thrown in the works. This can make it harder for your body to manage histamine, leading to the potential for high histamine symptoms. For example, chloroquine, which is used as an antimalarial drug, inhibits DAO production by 90%. Similarly, clavulanic acid, which is found in the antibiotic Augmentin, also inhibits diamine oxidase by 90%. Cimetidine, which is an H2 blocker, also decreases DAO production by about 50%. Acetylcysteine and amitriptyline both showed a slight inhibition of DAO.[62]

Additional drains on the DAO enzyme

The DAO enzyme is also used by the body to break down other biogenic amines including: tyramine, putrescine, cadaverine, spermidine, and spermine.

---

[61] Maintz et al., "Association of Single Nucleotide Polymorphisms in the Diamine Oxidase Gene with Diamine Oxidase Serum Activities."
[62] Leitner, Zoernpfenning, and Missbichler, "Evaluation of the Inhibitory Effect of Various Drugs / Active Ingredients on the Activity of Human Diamine Oxidase in Vitro."

High levels of other biogenic amines can reduce the ability of DAO to break down histamine. A recent research study found that high levels of putrescine or cadaverine could reduce the breakdown of histamine by DAO by up to 80%, while tyramine, spermidine, and spermine at high concentrations reduced histamine breakdown by up to 45%.[63]

Foods that contain high levels of tyramine include:

- Aged, smoked, or fermented meats
- Aged cheeses (cheddar, gouda, Swiss, parmesan, feta, Brie, etc.)
- Marmite and other yeasty things

Foods that contain spermidine and spermine include:

- Aged cheeses
- Hazelnuts, chicken liver, peas
- Soy-based foods

Note that there is a lot of overlap between foods that contain tyramine, spermidine, and spermine with foods that contain histamine. Essentially, limiting foods high in histamine will also cut down on other biogenic amines in your diet. You won't need to incorporate another diet or worry about food lists specific to the other dietary biogenic amines.

Gastrointestinal disorders and the production of DAO:
As explained above, the DAO enzyme is secreted by the cells lining the intestines into the intestinal mucosa to counteract histamine in food and histamine produced by the gut microbiome. Therefore, gastrointestinal disorders that affect the function of the cells in the intestines, such as celiac disease, IBS, or IBD, can reduce the production of DAO.

Histamine in the gut impacts gut motility, increasing motility through altering ion levels. One study explains: "Excess of histamine in gut lumen may trigger diarrhea, abdominal pain or constipation by increasing neurosecretory functions and muscle contractility."[64]

---

[63] Sánchez-Pérez et al., "The Rate of Histamine Degradation by Diamine Oxidase Is Compromised by Other Biogenic Amines," May 25, 2022.
[64] Neree et al., "Vegetal Diamine Oxidase Alleviates Histamine-Induced Contraction of Colonic Muscles."

We will dive into how the gut microbiome affects histamine levels in the next chapter.

Histamine N-methyltransferase (HNMT) Enzyme Production

The second way that the body controls histamine levels is by breaking it down with the histamine n-methyltransferase enzyme. The HNMT enzyme breaks down histamine throughout the body and is present in most tissues. HNMT is most abundant in the kidney, liver spleen, lungs, neurons, ovaries, and prostate gland.[65]

Histamine acts as a neurotransmitter in the brain, and HNMT is essential in regulating the level of histamine there. Neurons that respond to histamine are called histaminergic neurons. They are responsible for diverse physiological functions, including appetite, wakefulness, and memory. Genetic variants that change HNMT levels in the brain are linked to an increased risk of neurodegenerative disorders such as Parkinson's disease. Studies also link HNMT variants to an increased risk of migraines and ADHD.[66] Researchers have identified rare mutations in the HNMT gene that cause the enzyme to be inactive. These non-functioning mutations allow for too much histamine in the brain during neuronal development, which results in neurodevelopmental disorders, such as intellectual disability. [67]

In addition to breaking down histamine in the central nervous system, the HNMT enzyme acts throughout the body. HNMT is expressed in various tissues throughout the body, including the skin, lungs, and digestive tract, where it helps maintain histamine balance and prevents excessive inflammation.

---

[65] Shulpekova et al., "Food Intolerance."

[66] Yoshikawa, Nakamura, and Yanai, "Histamine N-Methyltransferase in the Brain," February 10, 2019.

[67] Heidari et al., "Mutations in the Histamine N-Methyltransferase Gene, HNMT, Are Associated with Nonsyndromic Autosomal Recessive Intellectual Disability."

One example of HNMT's significance in other tissues is its association with atopic dermatitis, also known as eczema. Atopic dermatitis is a chronic inflammatory skin condition characterized by itching, redness, and dry, cracked skin. A study by Kennedy et al. found that a specific variation in the HNMT gene was significantly associated with atopic dermatitis in children. This research highlights the role of high histamine levels due to decreased HNMT in developing atopic dermatitis.[68]

When histamine is degraded with the help of the HNMT enzyme, it forms N-methylhistamine, which is unable to bind to histamine receptors. The N-methylhistamine is further broken down with the MAO-B enzyme, forming N-methylimidazole acetaldehyde.[69] Important here is that a methyl group is needed in the reaction for breaking down histamine. We will come back to the role of methyl groups and the methylation cycle in just a bit because this can be an area to look at for optimizing your response to histamine.

Genetic variants that decrease HNMT enzyme production are linked to:

- ADHD and hyperactivity due to food additives.
- Asthma
- Eczema
- Migraines
- Alcohol use disorder
- Neurocognitive changes

If you have genetic data from 23andMe, AncestryDNA, or a similar service, you can check the raw data for the following HNMT variants:

[68] Kennedy et al., "Association of the Histamine N-Methyltransferase C314T (Thr105Ile) Polymorphism with Atopic Dermatitis in Caucasian Children."
[69] Maršavelski et al., "Why Monoamine Oxidase B Preferably Metabolizes N-Methylhistamine over Histamine."

Check your genetic data for **rs105089**:

- G/G: typical; lower risk of hyperactivity in ADHD due to food additives[70]
- A/G: reduced breakdown of histamine compared to G/G
- A/A: reduced breakdown of histamine compared to G/G[71]

Check your genetic data for **rs11558538**:

- T/T: reduced HNMT activity[72] higher histamine levels, increased relative risk of asthma[73]
- C/T: reduced breakdown of histamine, increased risk of asthma
- C/C: typical

Check your genetic data for **rs2071048**:

- T/T: increased risk of asthma (and higher histamine), common variant[74]
- C/T: typical asthma risk
- C/C: typical asthma risk

---

[70] Yoshikawa, Nakamura, and Yanai, "Histamine N-Methyltransferase in the Brain," February 10, 2019.

[71] Stevenson et al., "The Role of Histamine Degradation Gene Polymorphisms in Moderating the Effects of Food Additives on Children's ADHD Symptoms."

[72] Meza-Velázquez et al., "Association of Diamine Oxidase and Histamine N-Methyltransferase Polymorphisms with Presence of Migraine in a Group of Mexican Mothers of Children with Allergies."

[73] Raje et al., "Genetic Variation within the Histamine Pathway among Patients with Asthma."

[74] Raje et al.

Drugs that impair HNMT:

Similar to medications that decrease DAO activity, certain medications can also impact the way that the HNMT enzyme functions. According to research studies, medications that impair HNMT enzyme function include:[75]

- chloroquine
- amodiaquine
- tacrine
- etoprine
- metoprine
- chloroquine
- quinacrine
- dimaprit

Please be sure to talk with your doctor or pharmacist if you have questions about your medications.

Histidine Decarboxylase (HDC) Enzyme Production

The other half of the picture is the endogenous creation of histamine. The breakdown of histamine from food (DAO) and in the body (HNMT) balances out the production of histamine from histidine with the help of the HDC enzyme.

Histamine is made from the amino acid histidine. It is an essential amino acid, meaning humans cannot make it in our bodies and must obtain it from diet. Histidine can be used in the body for several different purposes, including histamine production.

Histidine decarboxylase (HDC gene) is an enzyme that catalyzes the reaction of histidine into histamine. It does this inside various cell types, including creating histamine in large amounts in mast cells.

---

[75] Yoshikawa, Nakamura, and Yanai, "Histamine N-Methyltransferase in the Brain," February 10, 2019..

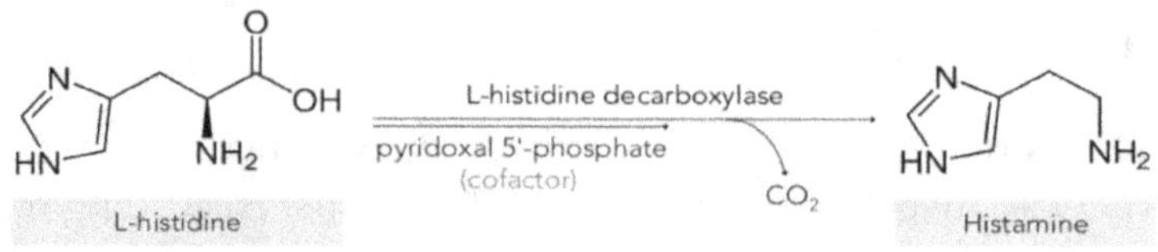

L-histidine conversion to histamine (from PMC7463562)

Not enough histamine:

Without enough histidine decarboxylase (HDC), animal studies show behavior that resembles Tourette syndrome. Histamine acts as a neurotransmitter in certain regions of the brain, and it also impacts other neurotransmitters, such as dopamine. Researchers have found that not enough HDC, due to rare genetic mutations, is one cause of disruption in the brain connection between histaminergic and dopaminergic neurons. Essentially, the decrease in histamine in the basal ganglia results in too much dopamine in that region of the brain, causing the tics seen in Tourette's.[76]

Animal studies also show that reducing the HDC enzyme (and reducing histamine production) causes changes to the way specific immune system cells behave. Macrophages are a type of immune system cell that can defend against bacterial infections as well as interact with the gut barrier. In mice with reduced HDC enzyme production, researchers found that the stomach lining changed in a way that caused chronic inflammation of the tissue. The researchers found that this was due to impaired maturation of macrophages, a type of immune system cell. [77]

Too much histamine and the heart:

Histamine is also essential in the way that the heart muscle functions. Too much histamine here can be detrimental, and people with chronic heart failure have higher average plasma histamine levels. In fact, a genetic variant in the HDC gene that reduces histamine production and overall histamine levels is linked to a significantly decreased risk of chronic heart failure.[78]

---

[76] Castellan Baldan et al., "Histidine Decarboxylase Deficiency Causes Tourette Syndrome."
[77] Kim et al., "Histamine Signaling Is Essential for Tissue Macrophage Differentiation and Suppression of Bacterial Overgrowth in the Stomach."
[78] He et al., "Relation of Polymorphism of the Histidine Decarboxylase Gene to Chronic Heart Failure in Han Chinese."

Additionally, clinical trials show that blocking the H2 receptor is beneficial for chronic heart failure. Famotidine improved cardiac symptoms and ventricular remodeling. In the heart, histamine increases the force of contraction, and even as far back as 1913, histamine has been known to induce heart arrhythmias.[79]

The HNMT enzyme's ability to break down histamine is heavily dependent on the availability of methyl groups. This is where the methylation cycle comes into play. In the following section, we'll explore how genetic variations in the MTHFR gene, a critical component of the methylation cycle, can influence the production of methyl groups and, consequently, the efficiency of histamine breakdown.

MTHFR and the Methylation Cycle

The methylation cycle is a biochemical pathway in cells that is involved in the generation of methyl groups. Methyl groups are used in many biological reactions. For example, serotonin is converted into melatonin in a reaction that uses a methyl group.

Important here: HNMT (histamine n-methyltransferase) incorporates a methyl group in the breakdown of histamine.

Chemically, a methyl group is a carbon attached to three hydrogens. It is a simple building block that can be added to other molecules to synthesize new substances. The methylation cycle is how methyl groups are generated and recycled for use in cells.

Folate, also known as vitamin B9, is a major player in the methylation cycle, serving as a primary source of methyl groups. When we consume folate-rich foods, dietary folate is converted into its active form, methylfolate. Through a series of biochemical steps, methylfolate interacts with vitamin B12 to generate methyl groups, which are then utilized in countless cellular reactions, including the crucial process of histamine breakdown by the HNMT enzyme.

---

[79] Kim et al., "Impact of Blockade of Histamine H2 Receptors on Chronic Heart Failure Revealed by Retrospective and Prospective Randomized Studies."

MTHFR genetic variants

Genetic variants in the MTHFR gene can reduce your production of methyl groups, especially in conjunction with a diet low in folate.

Two well-studied genetic variants are referred to as C677T and A1298C. Both variants reduce the functionality of the MTHFR enzyme, but the C677T variant causes a greater impairment.

About half the population carries one of these MTHFR variants, reducing their ability to convert folate into methyl groups. This is one of the most researched genes, with thousands of studies showing that decreased MTHFR function combined with not eating enough folate-rich foods can affect your susceptibility to many chronic conditions.

If you have genetic data from 23andMe, AncestryDNA, or a similar service, you can check for the following MTHFR variants:

Check your genetic data for **rs1801133**:

- G/G: typical
- A/G: one copy of MTHFR C677T allele (heterozygous) decreased MTHFR enzyme function by 40%[80]
- A/A: two copies of MTHFR C677T (homozygous) decreased enzyme function by 70 – 80%

Check your genetic data for **rs1801131**:

- T/T: typical
- G/T: one copy of MTHFR A1298C (heterozygous), slightly decreased MTHFR enzyme function
- G/G: two copies of MTHFR A1298C (homozygous), decreased enzyme by about 20%

---

[80] Choi et al., "The Association between MTHFR Polymorphism, Dietary Methyl Donors, and Childhood Asthma and Atopy."

Foods high in folate:

The US RDA for folate is 400 mcg per day of dietary folate equivalents (DFE). The DFE is a way of comparing supplements with folate to dietary folate. Essentially, supplemental folate (either methylfolate or folic acid) is considered a little more bioavailable than folate from foods. Getting plenty of folate-rich foods will provide the methyl groups needed to break down histamine in HNMT-catalyzed reactions. The NIH publishes the following information on natural folate sources in foods:[81]

Food	(mcg)/serving	% DV
Beef liver, braised, 3 ounces	215	54%
Spinach, boiled, ½ cup	131	33%
Black-eyed peas (cowpeas), boiled, ½ cup	105	26%
Asparagus, boiled, 4 spears	89	22%
Brussels sprouts, frozen, boiled, ½ cup	78	20%
Spaghetti, cooked, enriched, ½ cup†	74	19%
Lettuce, romaine, shredded, 1 cup	64	16%
Avocado, raw, sliced, ½ cup	59	15%
Spinach, raw, 1 cup	58	15%
Broccoli, chopped, frozen, cooked, ½ cup	52	13%
Mustard greens, chopped, frozen, boiled, ½ cup	52	13%
Bread, white, 1 slice†	50	13%
Green peas, frozen, boiled, ½ cup	47	12%
Kidney beans, canned, ½ cup	46	12%
Wheat germ, 2 tablespoons	40	10%

---

[81] "Office of Dietary Supplements - Folate."

Folic acid or methylfolate?

Supplemental folate is available as folic acid or methylfolate. If you don't regularly get the 400 mcg of recommended folate in your diet, you may want to consider supplementing to meet that need.

Folic acid is a synthetic form of folate that is added to fortified foods and some multivitamins. As a synthetic vitamin, it is a stable form that can handle the conditions involved in creating processed foods like cereal and pasta. However, folic acid must be converted into the active form needed in your cells, and this conversion process involves the MTHFR enzyme.

Methylfolate is the active form of folate and will bypass any problems in the MTHFR gene, making it easier for cells to produce methyl groups. Be sure to check the labels on methylfolate supplements as some brands contain high amounts of methylfolate, well above the 400 mcg/day RDA.

Talk with your doctor or health care provider if you have any questions about supplements or interactions with medications that you take.

Chapter 6: Gut Microbes Impact Histamine Levels

Key takeaways:

- Some bacteria in your gut microbiome make histamine, and other bacteria can limit histamine production.
- Balancing your gut microbes can go a long way toward relieving histamine-related symptoms.
- Many probiotics on the market contain histamine-producing bacteria, so choose your probiotics carefully.

In addition to histamine from dietary sources, the gut microbiome plays a major role in modulating histamine levels. For some people, histamine-related symptoms start or worsen when they focus on 'fixing the gut'. A lot of healthy gut advice begins with eating more naturally fermented foods, which can be very high in histamine as well as containing histamine-producing bacteria.

Think of your gut microbiome as a bustling city, home to a diverse community of bacteria, fungi, viruses, and other microorganisms, each playing a unique role in the city's ecosystem. Your gut microbes can make vitamins, neurotransmitters, fatty acids, gas, and other substances that can either contribute to your health or work against you.

The bacteria in your gut can also make and secrete histamine. However, not all types of bacteria secrete histamine, making the variability of the gut microbiome a key issue for people with histamine-related health problems.

Let's dive deeper into the role of specific bacteria in producing or degrading histamine.

Histamine from Bacteria in the Gut:

The histamine-producing bacteria can include your regular gut microbial inhabitants or bacteria you introduce through probiotics and fermented foods.

Histamine-producing bacteria:
Some bacteria possess the HDC gene, which enables them to produce histamine. This gene encodes an enzyme that transforms the amino acid L-histidine into histamine. In addition, some bacteria may also have specialized transporters that allow them to move histidine into the cell and export the newly synthesized histamine into the gut.[82]

Adding to the histamine burden, gut microbes can also crank out other biogenic amines that also need the DAO enzyme for metabolism. All told, this can add up to quite a lot of extra histamine, tipping some people over the edge into histamine reactions.

Just as histamine is an important signaling molecule in humans, bacteria can also use it as a signal to each other and to modulate the immune response. Researchers have found that patients with histamine intolerance have "a significantly higher abundance of histamine-secreting bacteria."[83]

While certain bacteria contribute to histamine production, others help regulate levels by breaking it down. Let's explore how these histamine-consuming bacteria help maintain a balanced gut environment.

Histamine consuming bacteria:
Also important is that some resident gut bacteria, such as *Pseudomonas putida,* can metabolize histamine and use it as a carbon source. This means that gut microbiomes containing more *P. putida* will have reduced histamine absorption from food.

P. aeruginosa, another Pseudomonas species, is an opportunistic bacterium that is often picked up in hospitals and can cause sepsis or bacteremia. *P. aeruginosa* is also able to grow using histamine as its "food". Recent studies indicate that the virulence of *P. aeruginoa* depends on access to histamine.[84]

---

[82] Mou et al., "The Taxonomic Distribution of Histamine-Secreting Bacteria in the Human Gut Microbiome."
[83] Sánchez-Pérez et al., "Intestinal Dysbiosis in Patients with Histamine Intolerance."
[84] Krell et al., "Histamine."

The picture that emerges is that the gut microbiome plays a critical role in balancing histamine-producing and histamine-degrading bacteria. An imbalance of these bacterial species could cause someone to have higher levels of histamine.

The gut microbiome in histamine intolerance:
A recent study shed light on the uniqueness of the gut microbiome in individuals with histamine intolerance. The findings showed significant differences in the gut microbiomes of people with histamine intolerance compared to normal gut microbiomes. In people with histamine intolerance, histamine-secreting bacteria were abundant, including *Staphylococcus*, *Proteus*, and *Enterobacteriaceae* species. Furthermore, the researchers identified high histamine-producing species *Clostridium perfringens* and *Enterococcus faecalis,* which can be pathogenic in people with decreased immune response. The researchers concluded: "A greater abundance of histaminogenic bacteria would favor the accumulation of high levels of histamine in the gut, its subsequent absorption in plasma and the appearance of adverse effects, even in individuals without DAO deficiency."[85]

The role of the gut microbiome is being studied to determine how histamine-producing bacteria may affect histamine-related conditions throughout the body. Further evidence of the gut microbiome's role in histamine levels comes from studies on inflammatory bowel diseases like Crohn's and ulcerative colitis. Researchers have found that people with IBD (Crohn's disease or ulcerative colitis) have higher than normal levels of histamine-producing bacteria and histamine in the colon. This was discovered in a study that looked at hundreds of different metabolites from the gut microbiome, with histamine being a key one. The researchers found that gut microbiome-derived histamine causes an increase in intestinal motility (e.g., diarrhea) by activating histamine receptors. Both Crohn's disease and ulcerative colitis patients had higher fecal histamine levels than healthy controls.[86]

[85] Sánchez-Pérez et al., "Intestinal Dysbiosis in Patients with Histamine Intolerance."
[86] Chen et al., "A Forward Chemical Genetic Screen Reveals Gut Microbiota Metabolites That Modulate Host Physiology."

The gut microbiome's influence on histamine levels may also impact conditions beyond the gut. A study showed that asthma patients had a much higher burden of histamine-producing bacteria in their gut. This suggests that high levels of histamine come from multiple sources, including the gut microbiome and basophil histamine production in the lungs, which may play a role in asthma.[87]

Another study involving people with histamine intolerance symptoms found that they had on average, a much lower abundance of *Bifidobacteria* in the gut and higher levels of Proteobacteria and *Roseburia* species. The phylum proteobacteria includes *Morganella morganii,* which is strongly linked to histamine secretion.[88]

Probiotics that Increase Histamine

Probiotic supplements are often recommended for fixing the gut. They can be a great asset to your gut health – or – they can work against you if they contain histamine-producing bacteria. When you go to buy a probiotic, you'll find a huge array of combinations and options. You'll need to read the labels carefully to see which strains are included.

My goal here is to give you the current science on how probiotics relate to histamine production. I'm not going to recommend any specific probiotics or even say that everyone with histamine intolerance needs a probiotic. Everyone is unique!

Histamine-producing strains:
These are some common probiotic strains known to produce histamine:[89] [90]

- *Lactobacillus diolivorans*
- *Lactobacillus reuteri*
- *Streptococcus thermophilus*
- *Lactobacillus saerimneri*

---

[87] Krell et al., "Histamine."
[88] Schink et al., "Microbial Patterns in Patients with Histamine Intolerance."
[89] Garai et al., "Biogenic Amine Production by Lactic Acid Bacteria Isolated from Cider."
[90] Thomas et al., "Histamine Derived from Probiotic Lactobacillus Reuteri Suppresses TNF via Modulation of PKA and ERK Signaling."

Histamine-neutral strains:
On the other hand, these strains have been found not to significantly
increase biogenic amine levels:[91]

- *Lactobacillus plantarum*
- *Lactococcus lactis*
- *Lactobacillus casei*
- *Lactobacillus bulgaricus*

Histamine-lowering probiotics:
Certain probiotic strains have demonstrated the ability to reduce
histamine levels in the gut. These beneficial bacteria may help restore
balance to the gut microbiome and alleviate histamine-related
symptoms.:[92]

- *Bifidobacterium infantis*
- *Bifidobacterium longum*

Another factor to consider with probiotics and histamine is D-lactate
production.

D-lactate-free probiotics:
One recommendation you may find online for histamine intolerance is to
try a D-lactate-free probiotic. Lactate is produced during anaerobic
metabolism and there are two forms of lactate: L-lactate and D-lactate.
Chemically, they are defined as enantiomers - or the same compound
with a different three-dimensional shape. L-lactate is the form produced
by your cells, such as when you exercise hard and your muscles produce
more lactic acid.[93]

D-lactate is produced by certain strains of bacteria, many of which are
involved in fermentation. Very high levels of D-lactate in the body can
cause D-lactic acidosis, which affects the central nervous system, causing
slurred speech and difficulty walking. This condition is rare and usually
occurs only as a complication of short bowel syndrome after surgery to
remove part of the small intestine.[94]

---

91 Bover-Cid and Holzapfel, "Improved Screening Procedure for Biogenic Amine Production by
Lactic Acid Bacteria."
92 Dev et al., "Suppression of Histamine Signaling by Probiotic Lac-B."
93 Pohanka, "D-Lactic Acid as a Metabolite."
94 Monroe et al., "Identification of Human D Lactate Dehydrogenase Deficiency."

D-lactate can also be broken down by certain bacteria and fungi, using the enzyme D-lactate dehydrogenase. Humans can also produce D-lactate dehydrogenase, although the research on this is scant and new. *Saccharomyces cerevisiae* is one yeast that can break down D-lactate.[95] For people with histamine intolerances, sticking to a D-lactate-free strain may help with reducing histamine levels.

Combining with vitamin B6:
In addition to the bacterial strains, vitamin B6 levels may also impact histamine production from probiotics. Taking vitamin B6 with your probiotic may affect whether the probiotic increases your histamine levels. Research shows that P5P, the active form of vitamin B6, is used by some bacteria in the reactions that produce histamine. Theoretically, adding a high dose of B6 could increase histamine production in the gut.[96]

---

[95] Stuivenberg et al., "In Vitro Assessment of Histamine and Lactate Production by a Multi-Strain Synbiotic."
[96] Bover-Cid and Holzapfel, "Improved Screening Procedure for Biogenic Amine Production by Lactic Acid Bacteria."

Case Study: The Busy Professional

Tyla is a 42-year-old mother of two young boys. She is a partner at an accounting firm and works approximately 50 hours a week. For most of her life she has led an active life and eaten a clean diet. She exercises 3 times a week doing High Intensity Interval Training with weights.

Recently she read about how improving your gut health is good for overall health, so she started eating a lot more fermented foods such as kimchi, sauerkraut, kombucha, and kefir. She was having a fermented food or beverage 2-3 times a day to improve her gut health. She also started eating a lot more avocados and loves a good charcuterie board. She drinks white wine with dinner only on the weekends. She eats out once a month with her family but doesn't eat fatty, fried foods, or junk food.

She has noticed that she is having more knee pain and waking up in the middle of the night to use the bathroom. She also noticed that she was waking up around 4 am and tossing and turning in bed a lot. This was causing exhaustion in the late afternoon and feeling fatigued.

She has a long history of seasonal allergies that she has noticed are getting worse as she has gotten older.

Tyla is very confused about why her health seems to be getting worse despite exercising regularly and eating an anti-inflammatory diet.

Using raw data from 23andMe and Genetic Lifehacks summary report, it was discovered that Tyla carried genetic variants for histamine breakdown in her intestines and clearance from her bloodstream.

Dietary Recommendations

- Low-histamine diet
- Avoid fermented foods such as kefir, kombucha, kimchi, sauerkraut
- Avoid alcoholic beverages for 3 months

Supplement Recommendations

- Combination product with quercetin dihydrate + vitamin C

- High quality multivitamin with optimal levels of vitamins B9, B12 and B6
- A bioactive curcumin supplement, which is anti-inflammatory, prevents histamine release from mast cells

Lifestyle Recommendations

- Circadian rhythm reset:
    - Go to bed before 12 am
    - No access to electronic devices 1 ½ hrs. prior to bed
    - Blue light blocking glasses after dinner
    - No bright lights in the evening after sundown. Switch to Edison/vintage bulbs
- Yoga - at least 3 times a week
- Mindfulness meditation in the morning and before bed for 10-15 mins to help deal with stress. Stress and irregular circadian rhythm can lead to inflammation which can affect histamine release and breakdown in the body.

Three months after starting the new regimen, Tyla is no longer waking during the middle of the night to use the bathroom. She is also not having knee pain and has noticed an increase in energy and less fatigue. Apparently, the night wakings to use the bathroom were due to a histamine reaction in her bladder.

Part 2: Solutions

Chapter 7: Dietary Changes to Lower Histamine Levels

Key takeaways:

- A low-histamine diet is a good tool for getting histamine symptoms under control.
- For some people with high histamine symptoms, a low FODMAPs diet may help.
- How you cook different foods can also make a difference in the amount of histamine.

Modifying your diet is one of the primary ways to manage high histamine symptoms. Histamine-rich foods are at the heart of histamine intolerance and can raise your overall histamine levels. While dietary sources of histamine are only part of the picture, high-histamine foods can often be the tipping point that pushes you over the edge and into histamine-related symptoms.

The goal of lowering your histamine levels with dietary changes is to understand which foods are most likely to cause histamine-related symptoms. For example, a low-histamine diet can help you understand how you feel without extra histamine - giving you a baseline. However, there's a fine line between doing what you can to reduce histamine in your diet and going overboard and obsessing over every bite. Fearing food reactions is no way to live life to the fullest, but you also want to be aware of how you feel after eating too many histamine-rich foods.

A Low-histamine Diet:

One of the most effective ways to manage high histamine symptoms is by adopting a low-histamine diet. By reducing your intake of histamine-rich foods, you can give your body a chance to reset and find relief from troublesome symptoms. Let's take a closer look at what a low-histamine diet entails.

Sticking to a low-histamine diet should show you within a few days to a week whether high-histamine foods are at the root of your histamine symptoms. As a general rule, foods that have undergone fermentation or aging processes tend to be higher in histamine. This includes foods like sauerkraut, aged cheeses, kimchi, natto, pickles, wine, and even sourdough bread. Processed meats, such as deli meats, sausages, pepperoni, and salami, can also pack a histamine punch. Even seemingly innocent vegetables like spinach can be surprising histamine culprits. Now, I know what you're thinking — a lot of these foods are part of a healthy diet. Don't worry, the goal isn't to eliminate them forever, but rather to be mindful of their histamine content and adjust accordingly.

Here is a list of common high-histamine foods:

Raw egg whites	Chickpeas
Blue Cheese	Lentils
Hard cheeses that are mature	Spinach
Dried meat (jerky)	Soybeans, edamame
Cured ham	Tomatoes
Most organ meats	Anything pickled
Processed meats	Bananas (when over ripe)
Smoked meat, BBQ	Citrus fruits
Anchovies	Chocolate
Fish (unless fresh caught)	Guava
Meat that isn't fresh	Kiwi
Seafood (unless fresh)	Pineapple
Buckwheat, malted barley	Strawberries
Walnuts, pecans	Nori, algae
Avocados	Cumin
Eggplant	Mustard seeds
Hot peppers	Soy sauce, vinegar

For a more complete list of histamine levels in foods, see the Appendix.

Some of these foods may not always trigger histamine reactions for you. One reason is that food processing conditions significantly impact histamine buildup, so you may react differently to certain brands. Finding which foods and brands work best will likely involve some trial and error.

The way certain fermented foods are made can make a difference in whether one brand works for you versus another. For example, most soy sauce is very high in histamine due to the fermentation process, but there may be exceptions depending on the type of bacteria used to ferment the soy. Research shows that certain bacteria can reduce the histamine content of soy sauce.[97]

Be aware that drinking alcohol can cause mast cells to release histamine. For some, this may cause flushing when drinking. But for people with histamine intolerance, even alcoholic drinks that are lower in histamine may still cause a reaction.[98] See Chapter 11 for more information about alcohol and histamine reactions.

While a low-histamine diet eliminates many healthy and delicious foods, it can be a useful tool when used temporarily.

Using a low-histamine diet to reset your system

Armed with the knowledge of which foods are high in histamine, you can now use a low-histamine diet as a powerful tool to reset your system. Lowering your overall histamine levels can help to down-regulate the production of histamine receptors and stop the over-reaction to histamine. Trying a low-histamine diet for a period of time can also give you a lot of insight into how histamine affects your body. However, it may not be a diet you want to continue long term. A low-histamine diet restricts many healthy foods you may enjoy, such as spinach, strawberries, and avocados.

Use a low-histamine diet as a tool to learn which histamine-containing foods bother you the most. You could also go back to it as needed for a short-term way to get histamine reactions under control.

In addition to a low-histamine diet, a low FODMAP diet may also help reduce histamine levels, especially for those with gut issues.

---

[97] Ma et al., "Ratio of Histamine-Producing/Non-Histamine-Producing Subgroups of Tetragenococcus Halophilus Determines the Histamine Accumulation during Spontaneous Fermentation of Soy Sauce."
[98] Zimatkin and Anichtchik, "Alcohol-Histamine Interactions."

Low FODMAPs diet: Histamine and gut problems

Another dietary approach that can be helpful for those with histamine intolerance is the low FODMAP diet. A low FODMAP diet eliminates foods that contain fermentable oligosaccharides, disaccharides, monosaccharides, and polyols (FODMAPs). This type of diet is often used to treat irritable bowel syndrome (IBS), and for many people, the diet improves symptoms. Interestingly, there's a connection between the low FODMAP diet and histamine levels that's worth exploring.

A study involving IBS patients revealed a strong link following a low FODMAP diet and reduced histamine levels. The researchers looked at the changes that occurred due to the low FODMAP diet by following IBS patients who were randomly assigned to either a low FODMAP or a high FODMAP diet.

The patients on the low FODMAP diet had significant improvements in symptoms, but without changes in breath hydrogen, which is often measured in IBS to determine bacterial overgrowth. Instead, the researchers found that urine metabolic profiling results showed that histamine levels were 8 times higher in the high FODMAP group compared to the low FODMAP group.[99]

Following a low FODMAP diet causes significant changes in the gut microbiome - reducing the bacteria that thrive on fermentable fiber. The change in the gut microbiome likely shifts away from histamine-producing bacteria. In addition, a low FODMAP diet also eliminates many high histamine foods, so some of the relief may be due to simply reducing histamine levels in the diet.

A low FODMAP diet eliminates marinated meats, processed meats, legumes, dairy products, yogurt, artichokes, asparagus, cauliflower, garlic, green peas, mushrooms, onions, sugar snap peas, high fructose corn syrup, honey, and most sugar substitutes. You can learn much more about the Low FODMAP diet at Monashfodmap.com.

I'll go more in-depth in Chapter 13 on the role of histamine in IBS.

____

[99] McIntosh et al., "FODMAPs Alter Symptoms and the Metabolome of Patients with IBS."

Gluten sensitivity and histamine intolerance

In addition to the low FODMAP diet, some people with histamine intolerance find relief by adopting a gluten-free diet. While the connection between gluten and histamine may not be immediately apparent, there's some interesting research that suggests a link between the two.

Anecdotally, some people find that a gluten-free diet helps their high histamine symptoms. A gluten-free diet changes the composition of the gut microbiome and generally reduces the amount of highly processed foods eaten. To test whether a gluten-free diet interacts with histamine symptoms, researchers looked at the overlap in symptoms between histamine intolerance and gluten intolerance. The study concluded that there was a significant overlap in symptoms and that a low-histamine diet may help people with gluten sensitivity.[100]

Another study looked at people who suffered from gastrointestinal disorders and migraines. The study participants were tested for serum DAO activity to see if they had reduced breakdown of histamine from food and gut microbes. The results showed low DAO levels in 90% of the migraine sufferers who met the criteria for non-celiac gluten sensitivity.[101]

Cooking Methods for Reducing Histamine

How food is prepared makes a big difference in histamine levels.

Histamine levels in raw foods can be quite different from those in cooked foods, and the method of cooking can significantly affect histamine levels. Long, slow cooking, such as smoking meat, can cause histamine to build up. A recent study found that frying and grilling tended to increase histamine levels in foods while boiling caused little change.[102]

---

[100] Schnedl et al., "Non-Celiac Gluten Sensitivity."
[101] Griauzdaitė et al., "Associations between Migraine, Celiac Disease, Non-Celiac Gluten Sensitivity and Activity of Diamine Oxidase."
[102] Chung et al., "Effect of Different Cooking Methods on Histamine Levels in Selected Foods."

It's important to keep in mind that as food starts to decompose, the levels of histamine and other biogenic amines begin to rise. The DAO enzyme breaks down both histamine and other biogenic amines. When there's an increase in the other biogenic amines, it depletes your DAO enzyme and can cause histamine levels to rise.[103]

Here are some tips for reducing histamine levels in your food:

- Avoid leftovers that have been sitting in the refrigerator for a few days. Instead, try putting your leftovers in the freezer and defrosting them when you want to eat them.
- Freeze meat when you bring it home from the store and thaw it quickly the day you eat it.
- Look for fish or seafood that says "frozen at sea" on the package.
- Smoked meats, such as BBQ pork or brisket, can contain very high levels of histamine. Sometimes it's worth it, and sometimes it's not... you decide.
- Foods cooked in a crock pot (low and slow) are more likely to be high in histamine.

Planning ahead can help to mitigate symptoms. For example:

- If you're eating out and don't know how fresh the meat is, take a DAO supplement or quercetin before you eat (more on these supplements in the next chapter).
- If you had pepperoni pizza for dinner (even while knowing you'll probably regret it), take an H2 blocker before bed to prevent heartburn.
- During pollen season, you may find that sticking to lower histamine foods can help reduce your allergy symptoms.

Also, consider how long you are going to cook the food. A crockpot (slow cooker) can be great for a busy family or working individuals, but slow-cooking meat all day can lead to higher histamine levels in the meal. Instead, a quick pressure cooker, such as an Instant Pot, can be a great way to make your favorite crockpot recipes quickly, without the day-long buildup of histamine.

---

[103] Sánchez-Pérez et al., "The Rate of Histamine Degradation by Diamine Oxidase Is Compromised by Other Biogenic Amines," May 25, 2022.

While cooking methods impact histamine levels, certain dietary patterns like fasting or keto may also increase histamine release.

Ketosis and Histamine Release

Keto diets and intermittent fasting are popular ways to eat, but they can lead to unintended consequences if you're focused on histamine levels.

The body switches to burning fat for energy when you fast (or go on a low-carb diet), a process called ketosis. Researchers have found that histamine levels increase in ketosis. Specifically, fasting causes mast cells in the intestines to release histamine, which travels to the liver. In the liver, histamine activates H1 receptors, which triggers the production of oleoylethanolamide (OEA). OEA signaling then promotes ketogenesis.[104]

Does this mean that everyone with histamine-related symptoms should avoid fasting or a ketogenic diet? I don't think so. But if you try intermittent fasting or keto and find that it makes your symptoms worse, it may be due to the activation of mast cells and the release of histamine. Again, everyone is unique, so while keto or fasting may not cause problems for everyone, it is something to keep in mind when looking at your symptoms.

---

[104] Misto et al., "Mast Cell-Derived Histamine Regulates Liver Ketogenesis via Oleoylethanolamide Signaling."keto

Chapter 8: Natural Supplements for Reducing Histamine

Key takeaways:

- Natural, readily available supplements may help reduce histamine levels throughout the body.
- Supplements can break down histamine or prevent too much histamine from being released from mast cells.

Now that we've explored the power of a low-histamine diet, let's dive into the world of natural supplements that can help you take your histamine management to the next level. In addition to natural supplements, I also want to encourage you to talk with your doctor about prescription medications that may also be helpful for your situation. Also, before starting any supplements, be sure to talk with your doctor or pharmacist about supplement interactions with any prescription medications that you're already taking.

Research studies clearly show that specific supplements can be impactful in mitigating histamine symptoms and preventing more histamine release. These supplements work in two different ways: by helping your body break down histamine more efficiently or by preventing histamine from being released in the first place.

Let's start by looking at supplements that can give your histamine breakdown a boost.

Supplements for reducing histamine levels:

As we talked about in earlier chapters, diamine oxidase (DAO) and histamine N-methyltransferase (HNMT) are the two enzymes produced by the body to break down histamine. Diamine oxidase is abundantly produced in the intestines to metabolize histamine from food before it is absorbed in the gut. It is the main enzyme studied by researchers for improving histamine intolerance symptoms.

Let's look at some specific supplements that fall into this category:

Diamine oxidase (DAO) enzyme supplements:
If you're looking for a little extra help in breaking down histamine from your food, diamine oxidase (DAO) supplements might be just what you need. These supplements are like your personal histamine-fighting sidekick, ready to jump in and break down histamine in your gut before it has a chance to enter your bloodstream and cause trouble. The key is to take them before a histamine-rich meal, so they can get to work right when you need them most.

Several studies have examined the efficacy of DAO enzyme supplements:

- A 2019 study found that symptoms of histamine intolerance significantly improved when DAO capsules were taken before meals. Symptoms included in the study were: abdominal pain, intestinal colic, bloating, diarrhea, constipation, nausea, belching, vomiting, postprandial bloating, dysmenorrhea, headache, dizziness, palpitations, and collapse.
- The study participants took DAO enzyme supplements before meals, up to three times a day. What is interesting about this study is that the participants had significant symptom improvements after two weeks of taking DAO, but the symptoms improved even more after four weeks of supplementation.[105] To me, this reiterates the idea that an overall reduction of histamine levels for a period of time will downregulate the histamine receptors, leading to less sensitivity.
- Another study found that DAO supplements helped people with chronic urticaria (itching). The study showed a significant reduction in itching scores after 30 days of supplementation with DAO before each meal.[106]

---

[105] Schnedl et al., "Diamine Oxidase Supplementation Improves Symptoms in Patients with Histamine Intolerance."
[106] Yacoub et al., "Diamine Oxidase Supplementation in Chronic Spontaneous Urticaria."

In addition to DAO supplements, there are a few natural food sources of this enzyme. For example, pea shoots are naturally high in the DAO enzyme. Pea shoots are the first several inches of the pea plant that come up from the seed. If you like to grow microgreens or have a garden, growing pea shoots is easy to do. Harvest the pea shoot seedling after it has grown several inches. You can add the pea shoots to a salad or smoothie – they taste just like fresh green peas.[107]

Vitamin B6 (pyridoxal-5'-phosphate, P5P, or pyridoxine):
As mentioned, DAO requires vitamin B6 as a cofactor, so ensuring adequate B6 levels is important. People who are deficient in vitamin B6 may have reduced production of DAO and research shows that improving vitamin B6 status (if deficient) increases DAO levels.[108]

Pyridoxal-5'-phosphate (P5P) is the active form of this water-soluble vitamin. You can find supplements for either vitamin B6 or P5P at most health food stores, so you can choose the option that works best for you and your histamine-fighting needs. Foods high in vitamin B6 include salmon, fresh tuna, eggs, milk, potatoes, and chicken. The RDA for vitamin B6 is 1.3 mg/day for adults, increasing to 1.9 mg/day during pregnancy.[109]

In addition, one study found that stacking P5P with supplemental DAO increased the ability of the gut to break down histamine. Note that this was an animal study, so this may not apply to everyone.[110] Not sure if you are getting enough vitamin B6? Cronometer.com is a free online app where you can track the foods you eat each day to determine the nutrient content, including vitamin B6, of most foods.

Vitamin C:
In addition to DAO and vitamin B6, another nutrient that may aid histamine breakdown is vitamin C, especially for those with suboptimal levels.

Let's take a look at a couple of the studies on vitamin C and histamine:

---

[107] Masini et al., "Pea Seedling Histaminase as a Novel Therapeutic Approach to Anaphylactic and Inflammatory Disorders."
[108] Martner-Hewes et al., "Vitamin B-6 Nutriture and Plasma Diamine Oxidase Activity in Pregnant Hispanic Teenagers."
[109] "Snapshot."
[110] Neree et al., "Vegetal Diamine Oxidase Alleviates Histamine-Induced Contraction of Colonic Muscles."

Aerobic exercise causes histamine to be released as a vasodilator, increasing blood flow to improve oxygen delivery to muscles. In a study of healthy adults, vitamin C before exercise reduced histaminergic vasodilation.[111]

Studies show that intravenous vitamin C reduces histamine levels in people with allergic reactions. However, in people with normal histamine levels, vitamin C didn't further suppress the levels.[112]

Some people feel they have reactions to ascorbic acid, the most common form of supplemental vitamin C, possibly because it is made from corn. Alternatives here would include food sources of vitamin C, such as blueberries or acai, which are low in histamine.

While breaking down histamine is important, preventing its release from mast cells is another key strategy in managing histamine levels. This is where natural mast cell stabilizers come in – they help keep your mast cells calm and less likely to release histamine. Let's explore some of the most promising natural mast cell stabilizers.

Natural Mast Cell Stabilizers

Mast cell stabilizers are compounds that prevent or reduce the release of histamine and other inflammatory mediators from mast cells. This stabilization of mast cells is critical in managing the symptoms of histamine intolerance or excessive histamine levels. Below are several natural supplements, backed by scientific research, that have demonstrated potential as mast cell stabilizers. I want to give you many options here so that you can choose what works best for your situation.

---

[111] Romero et al., "Effect of Antioxidants on Histamine Receptor Activation and Sustained Post-Exercise Vasodilatation in Humans."

[112] Hagel et al., "Intravenous Infusion of Ascorbic Acid Decreases Serum Histamine Concentrations in Patients with Allergic and Non-Allergic Diseases."

Luteolin:

Luteolin is a naturally occurring flavonoid found in herbs such as parsley and thyme. It has been reported to decrease mast cell mediator release. One study found that luteolin inhibits mast cells from being stimulated by activated T cells, suggesting a role in preventing histamine release in autoimmune diseases.[113] Animal studies show that luteolin inhibits IgE antibody-mediated (traditional allergy) release of histamine.[114] Thus, luteolin may also help reduce overall histamine levels in someone with seasonal allergies.

Quercetin:

Quercetin is another flavonoid superstar when it comes to keeping mast cells in check. Quercetin is found in many fruits and vegetables, and it has shown promise in animal studies for its ability to prevent the release of histamine and other inflammatory mediators from mast cells.[115] This supplement is gaining attention for its potential therapeutic effects in histamine-related disorders. It has one of the strongest inhibitory effects, preventing 80% of histamine release from stimulated mast cells.[116]

Side effects from luteolin and quercetin:

While these luteolin and quercetin supplements are generally considered safe at normal doses, I wanted to add a note here about a possible genetic interaction.

Luteolin and quercetin both interact with the COMT enzyme, which is a key enzyme in methyl group reactions including regulating the rate of breakdown of some neurotransmitters. About 20% of the population has a variation of the COMT gene that causes the enzyme to function more slowly. For these individuals, quercetin and luteolin could theoretically affect the rate of neurotransmitter metabolism and cause mood swings, irritability, or anxiety. Not everyone with slow COMT function will have side effects from luteolin and quercetin, but I wanted to mention it here in case you notice that you are irritable or anxious an hour or two after taking these supplements.

---

[113] Kempuraj et al., "Luteolin Inhibits Myelin Basic Protein-Induced Human Mast Cell Activation and Mast Cell-Dependent Stimulation of Jurkat T Cells."

[114] Kimata, Inagaki, and Nagai, "Effects of Luteolin and Other Flavonoids on IgE-Mediated Allergic Reactions."

[115] Gao et al., "Quercetin Ameliorates Paclitaxel-Induced Neuropathic Pain by Stabilizing Mast Cells, and Subsequently Blocking PKCε-Dependent Activation of TRPV1."

[116] Kaag and Lorentz, "Effects of Dietary Components on Mast Cells."

If you have genetic data, you can check to see if you have the COMT slow variant:

> Check your genetic data for **rs4680** (Val158Met):
>
> - G/G: fast (higher) COMT activity
>
> - A/G: intermediate COMT activity (most common genotype in Caucasians)
>
> - A/A: slow (40% lower) COMT activity[117] (Be alert for side effects, such as irritability, with quercetin and luteolin.)

Vitamin D:

According to research studies, mast cell stability is also impacted by vitamin D status. Studies in cell lines show that mast cells are more easily activated when vitamin D levels are low. The vitamin D receptor on mast cells helps prevent mast cell activation by inflammatory cytokines.[118]

In addition to vitamin D, certain fungal and herbal extracts have also demonstrated promising mast cell stabilizing effects.

Cordyceps:

One such extract is cordyceps mushroom, which has shown particular efficacy in preventing mast cell degranulation in the gut. Traditionally known for its use in Chinese medicine, animal studies show cordyceps mushroom extract prevents mast cell degranulation in the gut, a common trouble spot for people with histamine-related problems.[119] If you're not familiar with cordyceps, it's a fungus found in Asia that has been used medicinally for more than a millennium. You can find it as a powdered supplement or in capsules. The powdered form is mild in flavor and can be mixed into beverages such as a smoothie or coffee.

---

[117] Chen et al., "Functional Analysis of Genetic Variation in Catechol-O-Methyltransferase (COMT)."

[118] Liu et al., "Vitamin D Contributes to Mast Cell Stabilization."

[119] Han, Oh, and Park, "Cordyceps Militaris Extract Suppresses Dextran Sodium Sulfate-Induced Acute Colitis in Mice and Production of Inflammatory Mediators from Macrophages and Mast Cells."

Resveratrol:
Another popular plant-based supplement, resveratrol has a complex relationship with mast cells. While it inhibits prostaglandin formation by mast cells, it paradoxically increases TNF-alpha production at low concentrations.[120] However, this may not cause inflammatory problems for everyone. Another study showed that resveratrol inhibited mast cell activation in vitro.[121] The increase in TNF-alpha, an inflammatory cytokine, warrants caution when considering resveratrol for histamine intolerance in people who are dealing with chronic inflammation.

Euphorbia hirta:
Shifting to herbal medicines, *Euphorbia hirta* is an Ayurvedic herb that shows inhibition of mast cell degranulation in animal studies. Traditionally used for asthma, animal studies show that *Euphorbia hirta* extract significantly reduces mast cell degranulation.[122] Be sure to read reviews on *Euphorbia hirta* and check for any interactions with medications you take.

Chicoric Acid:
Chicoric acid, a compound found in echinacea and chicory, is another multi-faceted natural agent that inhibits mast cell activation and inflammatory mediator release. It also reduces the release of inflammatory mediators such as TNF-alpha, IL-6, and histamine, making it a multi-faceted agent against histamine intolerance.[123] Chicory is a traditional hot beverage, somewhat similar to coffee in taste. You can even find chicory combined with coffee if you are a coffee drinker.

---

[120] Shirley, McHale, and Gomez, "Resveratrol Preferentially Inhibits IgE-Dependent PGD2 Biosynthesis but Enhances TNF Production from Human Skin Mast Cells."
[121] Bilotta et al., "Resveratrol Is a Natural Inhibitor of Human Intestinal Mast Cell Activation and Phosphorylation of Mitochondrial ERK1/2 and STAT3."
[122] Parmar et al., "Amelioration of Anaphylaxis, Mast Cell Degranulation and Bronchospasm by Euphorbia Hirta L. Extracts in Experimental Animals."
[123] Lee et al., "Effect of Chicoric Acid on Mast Cell-Mediated Allergic Inflammation in Vitro and in Vivo."

EGCG in green tea:
One of the components that gives green tea its anti-inflammatory effects is the polyphenol EGCG. Epigallocatechin gallate (EGCG) has been shown in studies to suppress IgE receptor activation in basophils and mast cells.[124] EGCG is readily available as a supplement, or you can get EGCG by drinking green tea. Note that some people find that tea exacerbates histamine problems, so drinking a lot of green tea is something to approach cautiously to see how you react.

Palmitoylethanolamide (PEA):
The fatty acid palmitoylethanolamide, which interacts with the endocannabinoid system, has also demonstrated the ability to reduce mast cell degranulation. Several studies show that PEA may also reduce inflammation along with decreasing mast cell degranulation. One animal study found that PEA plus luteolin acted synergistically to reduce mast cell degranulation. Many of the animal studies with PEA focus on neuroinflammation and mast cells in the brain.[125] [126] This may be a good supplement to try if you experience mood shifts, pain, or cognitive symptoms from high histamine.

Curcumin:
Curcumin, the principal curcuminoid from turmeric, is well-known for its anti-inflammatory properties and has shown the potential to inhibit mast cell activation as well. For example, one study found that curcumin both decreased mast cell degranulation and suppressed the release of the inflammatory cytokine TNF-alpha release.[127]

Saffron:
Used since ancient times as a spice and medicine, saffron has been shown in animal studies to inhibit mast cell degranulation and reduce IgE allergic reactions.[128]

---

[124] Tachibana et al., "The Downregulation of Mast Cell Activation Through the Suppression of the High-Affinity IgE Receptor Expression by Green Tea Catechin Egcg."
[125] Lama et al., "Palmitoylethanolamide Dampens Neuroinflammation and Anxiety-like Behavior in Obese Mice."
[126] Parrella et al., "PEA and Luteolin Synergistically Reduce Mast Cell-Mediated Toxicity and Elicit Neuroprotection in Cell-Based Models of Brain Ischemia."
[127] Lee et al., "Curcumin, a Constituent of Curry, Suppresses IgE-Mediated Allergic Response and Mast Cell Activation at the Level of Syk."
[128] Lertnimitphun et al., "Safranal Alleviated OVA-Induced Asthma Model and Inhibits Mast Cell Activation."

Tulsi Tea or Holy Basil:
Turning to traditional beverages, tulsi tea or holy basil from India has
been found to inhibit histamine release and block mast cell degranulation.
The Latin name is *Ocimum tenuiflorum*, and it is also commonly called Holy
Basil. A 2016 study on *Ocimum tenuiflorum* found that it inhibits histamine
release and blocks mast cell degranulation.[129]

Targeting TRPV1

In addition to mast cell stabilizers, another therapeutic approach is to
modulate the TRPV1(transient receptor potential vanilloid 1) receptor
involved in histamine-induced itching and pain sensations. Although
histamine has been known for almost 100 years to cause itching, research
on how the signal for itching is transmitted to the brain is fairly new. The
TRPV1 receptor is located on peripheral nerves and interacts with
histamine to send the signal to the brain for pain or itching.[130]

The good news is that several natural supplements have shown promise
in targeting this receptor. If you're struggling with histamine-related
itching or stomach pain, these supplements might be worth exploring as
part of your symptom management plan.

Riboflavin:
Riboflavin, also known as vitamin B2, has been shown in studies to
modulate skin problems, such as itching and inflammation. In animal
studies, riboflavin reduces histamine-induced itching. New research
shows that riboflavin interacts with TRPV1 activity and prevents the
receptor from being overactivated by histamine.[131]

---

[129] Prakash et al., "Effect of Ocimum Tenuiflorum Linn Extract on Histamine Mediated Allergic
Inflammation in Human Mast Cells."
[130] Wilzopolski et al., "TRPV1 and TRPA1 Channels Are Both Involved Downstream of
Histamine-Induced Itch."
[131] Lee et al., "Riboflavin Inhibits Histamine-Dependent Itch by Modulating Transient Receptor
Potential Vanilloid 1 (TRPV1)."

Osthol:

A component of coumarin, osthol is a natural substance that modulates TRPV1 activity. It is found in Chinese herbal medicines such as *Cnidium monnieri*. Animal studies clearly show that osthol improves histamine-induced itching. Researchers have also found that Ostol reduces the activation of TRPV1 by histamine.[132]

---

[132] Yang et al., "Osthole Inhibits Histamine-Dependent Itch via Modulating TRPV1 Activity."

Chapter 9: Environmental and Lifestyle Factors

Key takeaways:

- We come in contact with chemicals and substances daily that cause histamine release from mast cells.
- Histamine acts as a vasodilator and is released with hard exercise.
- Motion sickness and vibrations can also cause histamine release.

We often think of histamine as something that comes from the foods we eat or the allergens we encounter, but did you know that there are countless substances in our everyday environment that can trigger histamine release from mast cells? For someone who doesn't degrade histamine all that well, these little exposures may add up - especially if combined with an environmental allergen or eating high histamine foods.

Let's dig into some of the research on substances that cause mast cells to release histamine.

Substances That Cause Mast Cell Degranulation:

Research studies show that quite a few common environmental chemicals and food additives cause mast cells to release histamine. The amount released is likely not a problem for most people, but for someone who has an excess of mast cells or a higher histamine burden, these may play a role.

Sodium fluoride:

Researchers have known for decades that sodium fluoride can trigger histamine release from mast cells. In one study, rats were given water with fluoride levels more than 20 times higher than what you'd find in your typical fluoridated municipal water system. The results showed that the animals had increased histamine levels in their brains, along with neuroinflammation.[133] Keep in mind that the levels used in this study were much higher than what you'd encounter in your daily life.

While the fluoride concentrations in fluoridated drinking water alone are unlikely to trigger much of a histamine reaction, it may be worth keeping an eye on how much fluoride you get daily if you regularly use fluoridated mouthwash and fluoridated toothpaste alongside fluoride in your water. Multiple sources of fluoride can add up, and fluoride does stick around in the body. A study on concentrated fluoride applied at the dentist showed that levels peaked after 60 minutes, declined over the next 20 hours, but were still detectable for three months.[134]

Research shows that N-acetylcysteine (NAC), an antioxidant supplement, increases the release of histamine from mast cells in conjunction with fluoride. Interestingly, the study did not show that NAC caused histamine release when paired with other known mast cell activators.[135]

PFOAs or PFAS:

Perfluorooctanoic acid (PFOA) is a class of chemicals used in many applications including non-stick pans and food packaging materials. A 2017 study in the Journal of Applied Toxicology found that PFOA exposure increased histamine release in the presence of an IgE allergen. Additionally, the PFOA exposure upregulated several pro-inflammatory cytokines. [136]

---

[133] Reddy et al., "Fluoride-Induced Expression of Neuroinflammatory Markers and Neurophysiological Regulation in the Brain of Wistar Rat Model."

[134] Talwar et al., "Fluoride Concentration in Saliva Following Professional Topical Application of 2% Sodium Fluoride Solution."

[135] Hong, Francker, and Diamant, "Effects of N-Acetylcysteine on Histamine Release by Sodium Fluoride and Compound 48/80 from Isolated Rat Mast Cells."

[136] Lee et al., "Association between Perfluorooctanoic Acid Exposure and Degranulation of Mast Cells in Allergic Inflammation."

Perfluoroalkyl substance (PFAS) is an overarching term for different PFOAs and perfluorooctane sulfonates (PFOSs). A 2019 study in Norway showed that PFAS levels were linked to the risk of asthma and allergies in teens. The adolescents who had total serum PFAS levels in the top 25% were more than 3 times as likely to have asthma. Additionally, teens in the top 50% of serum PFAS levels were more than twice as likely to have nickel allergy.[137]

Avoiding PFAS completely may not be possible, but there are ways to reduce your exposure. First, look for non-stick cookware that doesn't contain PFOAs or PFAS. Next, consider how often you dust and clean your home. A big source of PFOAs is the treatments put on carpets and furniture to resist stains as well as industrial-strength cleaners. Breakdown from these household materials then makes dust a big source of PFAS in the home.[138] Simply dusting regularly, vacuuming with a HEPA filter vacuum, and running a damp microfiber mop over the floor goes a long way towards reducing PFAS in the home.

Bisphenols (BPA, BPS):
BPA is a component of plastics and flexible vinyl. It is similar in structure to estrogens and can act as an endocrine-disrupting chemical. Exposure to BPA is ubiquitous, and studies show that about 95% of people have BPA in them at any given time. BPA at levels that are commonly found in people enhances histamine to be released from mast cells. Cell studies show that both higher levels of BPA and very low levels of BPA cause increased mast cell activation.[139]

Avoiding BPA altogether is difficult, but there are ways to decrease your exposure.

Common sources of BPA and BPS include:

- plastic water bottles
- teabags that contain plastic[140]
- plastic or lined food containers

[137] Averina et al., "Serum Perfluoroalkyl Substances (PFAS) and Risk of Asthma and Various Allergies in Adolescents. The Tromsø Study Fit Futures in Northern Norway."
[138] Savvaides et al., "Prevalence and Implications of Per- and Polyfluoroalkyl Substances (PFAS) in Settled Dust."
[139] O'Brien, Dolinoy, and Mancuso, "Bisphenol A at Concentrations Relevant to Human Exposure Enhances Histamine and Cysteinyl Leukotriene Release from Bone Marrow-Derived Mast Cells."
[140] Hernandez et al., "Plastic Teabags Release Billions of Microparticles and Nanoparticles into Tea."

- thermal printed receipts (some), especially when combined with hand sanitizer[141]
- drinking hot beverages, such as coffee, from plastic or disposable cups[142]

One route of BPA exposure that is especially important in children is through contact with dust. One estimate showed that dust contributed to about 10% of BPA exposure.[143] Dusting regularly and vacuuming with a HEPA filter can cut down on dust significantly.

Off-gassing and Sick Building Syndrome:
Chemicals that off-gas from new carpet or new furniture can cause histamine-related symptoms, such as rhinitis or skin itching. [144]

Mold and mycotoxins:
Mold spores and mycotoxins can cause mast cells to release histamine. For example, airway fungal infections can trigger mast cell degranulation. Mold spores are recognized by receptors called toll-like receptors (TLR) on mast cells. This can then trigger a cascade of hypersensitivity reactions.[145]

Glyphosate:
Glyphosate, a widely used herbicide, has been shown to cause mast cell degranulation in the airways. The research was done on mice that were exposed to glyphosate-rich air to replicate the exposure of farm workers.[146] Glyphosate can be found in low amounts on agricultural foods that have been sprayed with it, and in agricultural areas, glyphosate may be both airborne during spraying and in the groundwater. While avoiding glyphosate completely may be hard, a simple change would be to avoid spraying it around your home.

[141] Semerjian, Alawadhi, and Nazer, "Detection of Bisphenol A in Thermal Paper Receipts and Assessment of Human Exposure."

[142] Hananeh et al., "Exposure Assessment of Bisphenol A by Drinking Coffee from Plastic Cups."

[143] "Exposure of Children to BPA through Dust and the Association of Urinary BPA and Triclosan with Oxidative Stress in Guangzhou, China - PubMed."

[144] Ebbehøj et al., "Outbreak of Eczema and Rhinitis in a Group of Office Workers in Greenland."

[145] Kritas et al., "Impact of Mold on Mast Cell-Cytokine Immune Response."

[146] Kumar et al., "Glyphosate–Rich Air Samples Induce IL–33, TSLP and Generate IL–13 Dependent Airway Inflammation."

Methylisothiazolinone:
Methylisothiazolinone is a common preservative used in cosmetics, shampoo, and personal care products – and a common cause of contact irritation reactions. Animal research shows that methylisothiazolinone causes an increase in mast cells and eosinophils, which likely leads to allergy-type reactions.[147] Other animal research shows that exposure to methylisothiazolinone causes a persistent increase in mast cells in tissue.[148]

Food additives that cause histamine release:
Three very common additives to processed foods have been shown to cause histamine release: Sodium benzoate, carrageenan, and polysorbate 80.

Let's look at the studies:

- Sodium benzoate, a preservative in many packaged foods, has been shown to increase histamine release in people with asthma, allergies, and atopic dermatitis.[149]

- Carrageenan is used as an emulsifier and thickener in many food products, such as ice cream, non-dairy milk alternatives, and some deli meats. Researchers very commonly use it in animal studies to cause sterile inflammation and histamine reactions.[150] While carrageenan reliably induces mast cell histamine release when injected into mice, there isn't as much research on carrageenan causing systemic problems as a food additive. This could be dependent on intestinal barrier function. You may want to experiment and see if it is a problem for you.

- Polysorbate 80 is a surfactant found in medications, supplements, and some foods. It causes histamine release in some people, through non-IgE pathways.[151] Polysorbate 80 is found in ice

---

147 Arriaga-Gomez et al., "Repeated Vaginal Exposures to the Common Cosmetic and Household Preservative Methylisothiazolinone Induce Persistent, Mast Cell-Dependent Genital Pain in ND4 Mice."
148 Kline et al., "Repeated Dermal Application of the Common Preservative Methylisothiazolinone Triggers Local Inflammation, T Cell Influx, and Prolonged Mast Cell-Dependent Tactile Sensitivity in Mice."
149 Schaubschläger et al., "Release of Mediators from Human Gastric Mucosa and Blood in Adverse Reactions to Benzoate."
150 Xanthos et al., "Central Nervous System Mast Cells in Peripheral Inflammatory Nociception."
151 Mi et al., "Non-IgE-Mediated Hypersensitivity Induced by Multivitamins Containing Tween-80."

cream and pickles, and it is a common additive in medications. You'll find it called polysorbate 80 or Tween-80 on labels.

Exercise and Histamine Release:

Exercise causes both histamine and tryptase levels to naturally rise. Research shows this is both due to de novo formation and mast cell degranulation. This release of histamine and tryptase increases blood flow to the skeletal muscles during exercise, which is important for bringing more oxygen to the muscle cells.[152]

This is a normal response for most people, and the body can handle a certain increase in histamine and tryptase. However, some people with mast cell activation syndrome may find that exercise triggers a mast cell event.

When it comes to exercise and histamine release, it's all about finding your sweet spot. This is another one of those 'experiment and track it' situations: Keep track of your workouts and note any mast cell-related responses over the following 24 hours. It might take some trial and error, but with a little patience and persistence, you'll be able to dial in the perfect amount of exercise that minimizes mast cell degranulation. You may want to include mast cell stabilizers in your experiment to see if they are helpful before a harder workout.

From the gym to the open road, histamine can rear its ugly head in some unexpected places. If you've ever experienced motion sickness, you know firsthand how histamine can turn a fun adventure into a nauseating nightmare.

---

[152] Romero et al., "Mast Cell Degranulation and de Novo Histamine Formation Contribute to Sustained Postexercise Vasodilation in Humans."

Motion Sickness and Histamine:

Motion sickness refers to feeling nauseated due to perceiving motion. It can also include headache, salivation, reduced alertness, and cold sweats. Sea sickness is an age-old form of motion sickness, but motion sickness can also be triggered by car travel, roller coasters, and even video games. If you are prone to motion sickness, you can likely think of many other triggers.

Histamine plays a role in motion sickness, but it isn't the whole story here. Both the vestibular system in the inner ear and certain regions of the brain are involved in reconciling motion to visual stimulus. Researchers theorize that the sensory mismatch of visual stimulus with the motion sensed by the inner ear causes autonomic changes. Both the cholinergic and histaminergic systems are involved.[153]

Diphenhydramine (brand name Benadryl) is an H1 receptor blocker, and it is also sold as a motion sickness medication by the brand name Dramamine. Diphenhydramine is considered a first-generation antihistamine, which crosses the blood-brain barrier and often causes sleepiness. (Newer antihistamines don't cause drowsiness because they don't cross the blood-brain barrier to block histamine receptors in the brain.) Animal studies show that antihistamines that cross the blood-brain barrier are more efficacious for preventing motion sickness.[154]

High histamine levels are part of seasickness. A study showed that taking Vitamin C, which reduces elevated histamine levels, helps with suppressing the symptoms of seasickness.[155]

Ginger and hesperidin are natural, supplemental options for reducing histamine levels that have studies showing efficacy for treating motion sickness.[156]

---

[153] Zhang et al., "Motion Sickness."

[154] Tu et al., "Brain Activation by H1 Antihistamines Challenges Conventional View of Their Mechanism of Action in Motion Sickness."

[155] Jarisch et al., "Impact of Oral Vitamin C on Histamine Levels and Seasickness."

[156] Rahimzadeh et al., "Nutritional and Behavioral Countermeasures as Medication Approaches to Relieve Motion Sickness."

While there isn't direct research on a low-histamine diet helping with motion sickness, it may be worthwhile to avoid high-histamine foods before going into a situation that you know is likely to trigger motion sickness.

Vibration Causes Histamine Release

For some, exposure to vibrations can trigger itching or hives, a condition known as vibration urticaria. This can happen when using machinery that vibrates, like an orbital sander, or even when you're just trying to enjoy a leisurely bike ride down a washboard gravel road.

While it seems odd that vibration can cause hives in some people, researchers have discovered that a specific receptor on mast cells is the cause. For most people, the receptor is fairly resistant to mechanical shaking, but in some people, with genetic mutations, the receptor is more easily activated by repetitive shaking.[157]

Mast cells are located in areas of the body, like the skin and lungs, that are influenced by mechanical stretching. Researchers have found that a genetic variant in the ADGRE2 gene is linked to an increased risk of vibratory urticaria. The ADGRE2 gene encodes a cell adhesion protein on the surface of mast cells. It is thought that it acts as a mechanosensor in mast cells, increasing mast cell degranulation due to vibration.[158]

---

[157] Naranjo et al., "CRITICAL SIGNALING EVENTS IN THE MECHANOACTIVATION OF HUMAN MAST CELLS VIA P.C492Y-ADGRE2."
[158] Boyden et al., "Vibratory Urticaria Associated with a Missense Variant in ADGRE2."

Chapter 10: Over-the-Counter Medications

Key takeaways:

- Readily available, over-the-counter medications may help with histamine-related symptoms.
- Some common medications can block the DAO enzyme from working and cause an increase in histamine levels.
- Antihistamine medications are available that block the H1 receptor or the H2 receptor.
- Most of these medications just block the receptor and don't decrease the amount of histamine in the body.

Several over-the-counter medications block histamine receptors or impact histamine degradation. However, some drugs can interfere with, and decrease, DAO activity. Prescription medications are also available that interact with mast cell activation and histamine levels. Please talk with your doctor about the options available to you. While some over-the-counter medications can be a tool for managing histamine-related symptoms, it's important to be aware that some common drugs can actually work against you by interfering with your body's natural histamine-fighting defenses.

Let's take a closer look at some of the culprits that can decrease DAO activity and potentially exacerbate your histamine woes.

OTC Drugs that Decrease DAO Activity:

This is just a partial list of drugs that have known interactions with DAO. Talk with your doctor or a pharmacist if you need more information on the specific medications that you use. [159]

---

[159] Hrubisko et al., "Histamine Intolerance—The More We Know the Less We Know. A Review."

- Ibuprofen
- Acetylsalicylic acid (aspirin)
- NSAIDs
- Ambroxol

Over the Counter H1 and H2 blockers:

There are many options available to block the H1 or H2 receptors. These antihistamines work by blocking the histamine receptors, bringing temporary relief for histamine-related symptoms. However, it's important to note that most of these medications don't actually break down histamine; they just prevent it from binding to its receptors.

I like to think of antihistamines as one tool to combat high histamine symptoms that may be useful along with lifestyle and diet changes. For example, combining an OTC drug initially with a low-histamine diet may help to both reduce histamine levels and give immediate symptom release. Please be sure to talk with your doctor about medication interactions if you are on prescription medications.

When you read about H1 receptor blockers, you may see a specific medication referred to as a first-generation antihistamine or a second-generation antihistamine. The first antihistamines were developed more than 50 years ago, and they generally cross the blood-brain barrier and make people sleepy or less alert. The second-generation antihistamines came to market in the 1980s and don't cause drowsiness. While all of these over-the-counter medications are considered safe for short-term use, keep in mind that long-term use may have unknown health effects.

Antihistamines that target the H1 receptor:

Cetirizine (brand names Zyrtec and Allertec-D) is a non-drowsy antihistamine that acts on the H1 receptor. Recent research shows that repeated use of cetirizine can reduce the number of degranulating mast cells, essentially acting as a mast cell stabilizer.[160]

---

[160] Fujimura et al., "Cetirizine More Potently Exerts Mast Cell-Stabilizing Property than Diphenhydramine."

Fexofenadine (brand name Allegra) is another H1 receptor antagonist. Of note, fexofenadine and green tea use the same transporter. Drinking green tea or taking EGCG along with fexofenadine may reduce the effectiveness of the fexofenadine.[161]

Diphenhydramine (brand name Benadryl) is a first-generation antihistamine that crosses the blood-brain barrier and makes people a little sleepy or less alert. Diphenhydramine also has anticholinergic properties, which makes long-term use in older adults a risk factor for dementia.[162]

Loratadine (brand name Alavert, Claritin) is another OTC option for a second-generation antihistamine that blocks the H1 receptor. Loratadine also has been shown to inhibit inflammation caused by advanced glycation end products. Specifically, one study found that it helped with inflammation in the connective tissue, such as in arthritis, by stopping advanced glycation end products from activating inflammation.[163]

Levocetirizine (brand name Xyzal) is a second-generation antihistamine that works as an inverse agonist to decrease the activity of the H1 receptors. Similar to cetirizine, it acts as a mast cell stabilizer to reduce degranulation.[164]

Now that we've covered the H1 receptor blockers, let's shift our focus to their counterparts: the H2 blockers.

H2 receptor blockers:

Over-the-counter medications that block the H2 receptor are mainly marketed for heartburn or GERD symptoms. This is because blocking the H2 receptor reduces stomach acid secretion by 70% over a 24-hour period. The effects are mainly on basal stomach acid secretion at night or during fasting.[165]

---

161 Misaka et al., "Exposure of Fexofenadine, but Not Pseudoephedrine, Is Markedly Decreased by Green Tea Extract in Healthy Volunteers."

162 Gray et al., "Cumulative Use of Strong Anticholinergics and Incident Dementia."

163 Gao and Zhang, "Loratadine Alleviates Advanced Glycation End Product-Induced Activation of NLRP3 Inflammasome in Human Chondrocytes."av

164 Fujimura et al., "Cetirizine More Potently Exerts Mast Cell-Stabilizing Property than Diphenhydramine."

165 "Histamine Type-2 Receptor Antagonists (H2 Blockers)."

Cimetidine (brand name Tagamet) was the first H2 blocker approved for use in the US in 1977. It is available as a prescription in doses of 300 to 400 mg, and it is also available OTC in doses of around 200 mg. Chronic use of cimetidine is linked to minor elevations in liver enzymes in 1-4% of people, which usually resolves after discontinuation. Note that cimetidine has been shown to reduce the production of the DAO enzyme.[166]

Famotidine (brand name Pepcid) is also available both OTC and as a prescription. Over-the-counter dosages are usually 10 to 20 mg, while prescription dosages are usually 20 to 40 mg. Chronic use of famotidine is also associated with elevated liver enzymes in 1 - 4 % of people.

Nizatidine (brand name Axid-AR) is a third option for an H2 blocker. Like famotidine and cimetidine, nizatidine is available in OTC and prescription doses. It also is linked to elevated liver enzymes in 1-4% of people.[167]

If you have liver or kidney disease, please be sure to check with your doctor before regularly using any of these H2 blockers.

Ranitidine (brand name Zantac) was previously available as an OTC medication but is no longer available in the US, EU, or Australia. A few years ago, it was discovered that ranitidine can break down and contain trace amounts of NDMA, a known carcinogen. As a result, ranitidine products were pulled from the market, and a stark reminder that seemingly harmless medications and supplements can have unknown risks.

---

[166] Leitner, Zoernpfenning, and Missbichler, "Evaluation of the Inhibitory Effect of Various Drugs / Active Ingredients on the Activity of Human Diamine Oxidase in Vitro."
[167] "Histamine Type-2 Receptor Antagonists (H2 Blockers)."

Chapter 11: Alcohol and Histamine

Key takeaways:

- Drinking alcohol is often a problem for people with histamine intolerance.
- Two different genetic pathways are at play here: histamine degradation and/or alcohol metabolism pathways.
- Understanding these pathways may help people with histamine sensitivity avoid alcohol-induced reactions.

Alcohol and its relationship with histamine represent a complex interplay that can significantly impact individuals with histamine-related reactions. This chapter explores the mechanisms by which alcohol affects histamine levels, the role of genetics, and practical strategies for managing these interactions.

As we dive deeper into the specific mechanisms by which alcohol can send your histamine levels soaring, you will discover that it's a perfect storm of histamine-boosting factors. Understanding these pathways can be key to managing your histamine-related reactions.

How Alcohol Increases Histamine Levels

Alcohol can trigger histamine reactions through multiple pathways, which can combine together to raise your histamine levels:

- Most alcoholic beverages contain histamine, which can provoke reactions in those with poor histamine degradation capabilities.
- The conversion of alcohol into acetaldehyde can stimulate histamine release.
- Alcohol impedes the DAO enzyme responsible for histamine breakdown.

Histamine in Alcoholic Beverages:

Alcohol is made through the fermentation of different grains or fruits, and histamine or other biogenic amine levels are typically high in fermented drinks. For instance, wine is often high in biogenic amines, including histamine. The level of histamine depends on the bacterial strains used in fermentation, so some wines are extremely high in histamine while others may not cause quite as many problems.[168]

Wine isn't the only alcohol with histamine in it, though. A 2009 study found histamine in all the beers that were tested.[169] While distilled spirits, such as whiskey and vodka, are generally lower in histamine than wine, reactions to distilled spirits are still common.[170]

Alcohol and DAO Inhibition:

Alcohol interacts with histamine production and histamine clearance in a couple of important ways.

First, when you consume alcohol, it partially inhibits DAO's ability to do its job. So, if you're already struggling with low DAO levels and having trouble breaking down histamine from food, adding alcohol to the equation is like pouring gasoline on a fire. It amplifies the issue and can lead to a build-up of histamine in your system.

Second, alcohol and acetaldehyde can directly trigger histamine release from basophils and mast cells in the periphery. This means that they can trigger histamine in the skin causing flushing, itching, and hives.[171] If you've ever flushed or gotten itchy after drinking, histamine release due to acetaldehyde is likely the cause.

---

[168] Regecová et al., "Detection of Microbiota during the Fermentation Process of Wine in Relation to the Biogenic Amine Content."

[169] Tang et al., "Determination of Biogenic Amines in Beer with Pre-Column Derivatization by High Performance Liquid Chromatography."

[170] Adams and Rans, "Adverse Reactions to Alcohol and Alcoholic Beverages."

[171] Zimatkin and Anichtchik, "Alcohol-Histamine Interactions."

Alcohol Metabolism and Acetaldehyde:
Alcohol goes through a multistep process to be broken down and eliminated by the body. Alcohol is first metabolized into acetaldehyde, which is then converted into acetic acid. Genetic variants in the enzymes responsible for this process (ADH and ALDH genes) can lead to acetaldehyde building up if it isn't converted quickly enough into acetic acid. The buildup of acetaldehyde further triggers histamine release from mast cells.[172]

Strategies for Managing Histamine Reactions to Alcohol:
The obvious solution here is to avoid drinking alcohol altogether. This can be easier said than done for many people, especially if social or work situations involve alcohol consumption.

One thing to try is eating a low-histamine diet on days that you know you are going to consume alcohol, which may help to avoid high histamine symptoms. If you're heading out to happy hour with colleagues or a party with friends, consider eating something ahead of time that you know won't cause a histamine reaction. Then when you're out having fun, you won't be as tempted by the high-histamine cheese tray or appetizers. Everyone is unique in their response to alcohol, though, so you may find that a low-histamine diet that day is not enough to mitigate your symptoms.

Opting for low-histamine alcoholic beverages may also help. Instead of wine, consider a fruity drink that contains a splash of a low-histamine alcohol, such as vodka or gin.

Supplements that may help when drinking alcohol:

If you're planning on indulging in a few cocktails, go prepared with supplements that can help to break down histamine or inhibit mast cell degranulation.

- DAO enzyme supplements can assist in breaking down histamine in alcoholic beverages.
- Quercetin and fisetin inhibit mast cell degranulation, reducing histamine release.

---

[172] Zimatkin and Anichtchik.

- Luteolin demonstrates potential in inhibiting histamine release from mast cells.
- MitoQ is a CoQ10-derived supplement that has been shown to enhance acetaldehyde clearance in the liver.[173]

---

[173] Hao et al., "Mitochondria-Targeted Ubiquinone (MitoQ) Enhances Acetaldehyde Clearance by Reversing Alcohol-Induced Posttranslational Modification of Aldehyde Dehydrogenase 2."

Part 3: A Detailed Look at Histamine-Related Conditions

Chapter 12: Histamine in the Brain

Key takeaways:

- Histamine acts as a neurotransmitter in the brain and it also modifies other neurotransmitters.
- Histamine levels are lower at night and rise in the early morning, which increases alertness and wakefulness.
- High histamine levels can play a role in migraines, neuroinflammation, mood disorders, and other neurological disorders.

Histamine plays several important roles in the brain. It acts as a neurotransmitter, sending signals between neurons, and acts as part of the innate immune response. As a neurotransmitter, histamine is involved in learning, attention, memory, and wakefulness. Histamine is produced within neurons and then broken down via HNMT in neurons and astrocytes. The histaminergic neurons are active during the daytime when you're awake, and they are not active during sleep.[174]

Animal studies show that histamine is one of the first neuromodulators found in developing embryo brains. Histamine receptors (H1, H2, and H3) are found throughout the developing brain regions. Studies also show that histamine plays a central role in the formation of neurons and neuronal circuits in the basal ganglia and striatum. Specifically, histamine is important in the differentiation of neuronal stem cells into GABAergic neurons.[175]

Let's look at a few of the ways that histamine in the brain impacts your everyday life.

---

[174] Takahashi, Lin, and Sakai, "Neuronal Activity of Histaminergic Tuberomammillary Neurons During Wake–Sleep States in the Mouse."
[175] Carthy and Ellender, "Histamine, Neuroinflammation and Neurodevelopment."

Migraines and High Histamine:

People with migraines understand that it is more than just a headache, affecting your whole body. Migraines are a complex disorder characterized by intense headaches often accompanied by nausea, vomiting, sensitivity to light and sound, and brain fog. While the exact causes are still being uncovered, research points to a key role of neurogenic inflammation.

Neurogenic inflammation refers to inflammation triggered by nerve activation. In migraines, stimulation of specific neurons or receptors leads to the release of pro-inflammatory neuropeptides. These neuropeptides initiate a cascade of inflammatory response including activating mast cells.[176]

Mast cells are found in the area around the sensory neurons that detect pain. Research studies clearly show that high histamine levels can trigger migraines or headaches, however, the studies are less clear as to whether H1 or H2 blocking medications have much of an effect. Interestingly, drugs that act on the H3 receptor and increase histamine levels in the brain have a known side effect of causing headaches.[177]

One key pathway in migraines involves the trigeminal nerve, a large cranial nerve that spans from the temple to the nose, eyes, teeth, and jaw. It is thought to play a central role in migraines. The trigeminal nerve can release pro-inflammatory neuropeptides that increase vasodilation.

Studies show that there is bi-directional communication between the sensory nerves and mast cells. In other words, the neuropeptides released can activate mast cells, and the histamine and serotonin released from mast cells can activate the trigeminal nerve.[178]

---

[176] Malhotra, "Understanding Migraine."
[177] Worm, Falkenberg, and Olesen, "Histamine and Migraine Revisited."
[178] Guan, Dong, and Green, "Roles of Mast Cells and Their Interactions with the Trigeminal Nerve in Migraine Headache."

Trigeminal Nerve

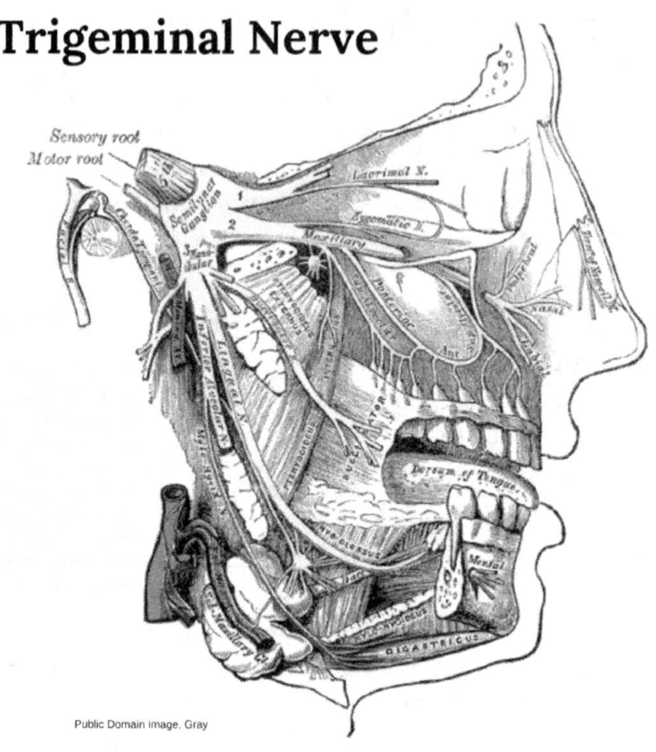

Figure 1: The trigeminal nerve extends across the face and head, with branches reaching the temples, eyes, nose, and jaw. Activation of this nerve plays a central role in migraine pathology. (Image: Public domain).

Neuroinflammation

Neuroinflammation is a general term for activating the brain's immune system – e.g., brain inflammation. Microglia are specialized immune cells in the brain that respond to infections or damage by releasing inflammatory molecules. They are the primary type of immune cell in the brain and throughout the central nervous system. They can react to infections or injuries, and activated microglia produce inflammatory cytokines to fight off pathogens.[179]

---

[179] Rock et al., "Role of Microglia in Central Nervous System Infections."

Neuroinflammation, often involving the activation of microglia, is increasingly recognized as a contributor to various neurological disorders. Surgery or injury is one way of triggering neuroinflammation and many people have postoperative cognitive dysfunction following surgery. Research studies show that neuroinflammation from surgery activates mast cells on microglia, leading to cognitive problems in the days after the procedure.

For example, researchers studied the post-surgery cognitive changes in animals to learn more about the molecular pathways involved. They found that mast cells are activated on microglia in the brain after surgery, as well as elsewhere in the body. Importantly, using mast cell stabilizers before surgery prevented neuroinflammation and memory dysfunction in the days after surgery.[180]

Injury and surgery are just one cause of neuroinflammation. Exposure to toxins or heavy metals can also cause inflammation, as can a viral or bacterial infection. While mast cell activation and histamine release are only part of what goes on in the inflamed brain, you may find that reducing your overall histamine levels improves brain function.

Neurological Disorders that Interact with Histamine

In the brain, microglial activation and neuroinflammation are associated with neurological disorders. All four types of histamine receptors are expressed on microglia, and histamine binding to the H1 and H4 receptors can cause microglia to secrete inflammatory cytokines, including TNF-alpha and IL-6. However, activation of H3 receptors on microglia moderates the inflammatory response. There is still more to learn on how altered levels of histamine in the brain can lead to microglial activation and neuroinflammation.[181]

---

[180] Zhang et al., "Activated Brain Mast Cells Contribute to Postoperative Cognitive Dysfunction by Evoking Microglia Activation and Neuronal Apoptosis."
[181] Carthy and Ellender, "Histamine, Neuroinflammation and Neurodevelopment."

Interaction with autism spectrum disorder:
Epidemiological studies show that there is a correlation between atopic disorders (eczema, allergies, asthma, and food intolerances) in infancy and autism spectrum disorder. Atopic disorders are strongly linked to high histamine levels from mast cell activation. While the mechanisms are still unclear, some researchers propose that disruption of the blood-brain barrier and activation of mast cells are involved in autism.[182]

I want to emphasize that it is still theoretical as to exactly how or why high histamine levels and mast cell activation could play a role in autism spectrum disorder (ASD). To help sort out if there is a causal role, the link between atopic disorders and autism spectrum disorder has recently been looked at using a Mendelian randomization study. This type of analysis uses known genetic connections to determine whether there is a causal association in a correlation. In this case, Mendelian randomization supports a causal link between atopic disorders and ASD.[183] More research is needed here to understand the complex pathways involved.

ADHD and high histamine:
Histamine in the brain can also be a factor in ADHD (attention deficit hyperactivity disorder). Genetic studies show that variants in the HNMT gene increase the susceptibility to ADHD. HNMT codes for the histamine N-methyltransferase enzyme which breaks down histamine throughout the brain. HNMT function is essential for the breakdown of histamine in the brain where it is used as a neurotransmitter.[184]

Artificial food coloring, additives, and processed foods have been shown to worsen ADHD symptoms and increase aggressive behavior in some individuals with HNMT genetic variants. Eliminating food coloring is often recommended for ADHD, and it may specifically help individuals with high histamine and HNMT variants.

Allergic rhinitis is the itchy, watery eyes and runny nose that occurs with seasonal allergies. Histamine release is the cause of the symptoms, and people often use over-the-counter antihistamine medicines for it.

---

[182] Theoharides et al., "Atopic Diseases and Inflammation of the Brain in the Pathogenesis of Autism Spectrum Disorders."
[183] Cao et al., "Causal Relationships between Atopic Dermatitis and Psychiatric Disorders."
[184] Yoshikawa, Nakamura, and Yanai, "Histamine N-Methyltransferase in the Brain," February 10, 2019.

A study involving children with allergic rhinitis and ADHD showed that treating their allergic rhinitis with antihistamines and nonpharmacologic interventions also improved their ADHD symptom scores.[185]

Collectively, these studies suggest that higher brain histamine levels, whether due to genetic differences in histamine breakdown or allergic triggers, may worsen ADHD symptoms in some individuals. Lowering high histamine levels may be beneficial for managing ADHD symptoms.

Depression and Anxiety:

Depression and anxiety are complex issues with multiple causes. High histamine levels are linked in multiple ways to depression and anxiety, but histamine isn't the only root cause of mood disorders. There are multiple pathways involved in depression and anxiety.

Research points to histamine in the brain interacting with other neurotransmitters, including serotonin and norepinephrine, to modulate mood. For example, activation of the H3 receptor in certain brain regions inhibits serotonin signaling and alters dopamine signaling.[186] Alterations in this delicate balance, as well as other factors like poor sleep and high-histamine diets, may contribute to mood imbalances in some individuals (see Case Study).

A study of teens with major depressive disorder found that the only significant difference in the depressed patients compared to a healthy control group was that histamine levels were about 25% higher in the depressed group. About 80% of the adolescents with depression also had food intolerances along with high serum histamine levels.[187]

---

[185] Yang et al., "Attention-Deficit/Hyperactivity Disorder-Related Symptoms Improved with Allergic Rhinitis Treatment in Children."
[186] Qian et al., "Histamine and Histamine Receptors."
[187] Tao, Fu, and Xiao, "Chronic Food Antigen-Specific IgG-Mediated Hypersensitivity Reaction as A Risk Factor for Adolescent Depressive Disorder."

It is hard to measure histamine levels in the brains of living people, but post-mortem samples can shed a lot of light on what is going on in the brain. A post-mortem analysis of brain cortex tissue compared histamine-related enzymes in people who had depressive disorders to healthy controls. The results showed that levels of HDC, the enzyme that converts histidine to histamine, were the same in depressed brains vs. normal. However, the levels of HNMT, the enzyme that breaks down histamine, were lower in the depression group. This would indicate normal production of histamine, but with less degradation, overall histamine levels were likely to be higher.[188]

The immune system and inflammation can also cause depressive symptoms. With the role of histamine in neuroinflammation, it is not surprising that activation of the histamine receptors in the microglia can increase inflammatory cytokines in the brain. Animal studies show that antihistamines that block the H1 receptor or the H3 receptor seem to alleviate depressive behavior, but human clinical trials are lacking here.

Balance is again an important theme here. Animal studies also point to low histamine levels in certain brain regions causing decreased activity levels, less alertness, and more depression-like symptoms.[189]

Animal studies also show that histamine levels are likely important in anxiety. Again, the H3 receptor in certain brain regions seems to play a key role through interacting with glutamine in the prefrontal cortex.[190]

Antihistamines have historically been used in pediatric and adult patients with generalized anxiety disorder. Hydroxyzine is a prescription H1 receptor blocker that has been used since the 1950s. It is a central-acting antihistamine, meaning that it can cross the blood-brain barrier and may make people sleepy. Research shows that it is effective in the treatment of generalized anxiety disorder without adverse side effects.[191]

Again, I want to make clear that major depressive disorder and anxiety disorders have multiple root causes. High histamine levels may play a role for some people, but not for everyone.

---

188 Shan et al., "Unaltered Histaminergic System in Depression."
189 Qian et al., "Histamine and Histamine Receptors."
190 Zhang et al., "Targeting Presynaptic H3 Heteroreceptor in Nucleus Accumbens to Improve Anxiety and Obsessive-Compulsive-like Behaviors."
191 Strawn et al., "Pharmacotherapy for Generalized Anxiety Disorder in Adults and Pediatric Patients."

Case Study: Lonely and Depressed

Bryan is a 20-year-old male with a long history of anxiety and depression. He started having difficulties with school in grade 6. He was diagnosed with ADHD and anxiety in grade 2 and was started on medication in grade 4. Much of the issues in elementary school were due to aggressive behavior towards his peers on the playground. In grade 10 his social anxiety and depression got so bad that he had to drop out of school. He currently doesn't leave the house due to the state of his mental health. He is neither working nor in school. His main goal is to be able to go back to school and get his high school diploma.

He has always had difficulties falling asleep and would often wake several times during the night. He has a history of asthma and nasal congestion. The nasal congestion has gotten progressively worse over the years, and it was affecting his sleep. In general, he tends to have a difficult time falling asleep and will often spend the night tossing and turning.

He has been diagnosed with Type II diabetes and obesity.

His genomic summary report revealed that he had variants that affected methylation, and histamine clearance systemically and in the digestive tract. He also has several inflammatory SNP's (single nucleotide polymorphisms) and decreased Bifidobacterium population in the gut microbiome.

Dietary Recommendations

- Low-histamine diet for 4 weeks to help clear out high histamine levels and reset
    - Avoid fermented foods such as kimchi, sauerkraut, kombucha, kefir since these increase histamine in the digestive tract
    - Eliminate artificial coloring, additives, and processed foods from the diet

- These have been shown to worsen ADHD symptoms and increase aggressive behavior in some individuals
- Eat a whole foods diet that is high in colorful fruits and vegetables
  - In particular, green leafy vegetables contain folate which can help improve the methylation cycle
- No eating 3 hours before bed

Supplement Recommendations

- Active Curcumin supplement to help manage inflammation
- Bifidobacterium only probiotic without prebiotics
- B complex - to improve methylation pathway
- L theanine - inhibits histamine release from mast cells and blocks glutamate activity in the brain
  - This is helpful to regulate the sleep/wake cycle
- Magnesium glycinate to stabilize the COMT gene, help decrease histamine levels in the body and act as a relaxing sleep aid

Lifestyle Recommendations

- Maintain a regular sleep/wake cycle
- Go to bed and wake up at the same time everyday
- Blue light blocking glasses after eating dinner

Chapter 13: IBS, Acid Reflux, and Histamine

Key takeaways:

- Histamine activates H2 receptors in the stomach to cause the release of stomach acid.
- High histamine levels in the gut may cause IBS symptoms including gastrointestinal pain.

Histamine is an essential signaling molecule in the stomach that triggers the release of stomach acid. However, too much histamine can cause problems with acid reflux or GERD. Similarly, too much histamine from mast cell activation or the gut microbes in the intestines can cause abdominal pain and bloating. H1, H2, and H4 receptors are present throughout the gastrointestinal tract. H4 receptors are present on intestinal mast cells as well as in the duodenum, colon, and mucosa. H4 receptors play a key role in the intestinal inflammatory response in colitis, allergic reactions, and irritable bowel syndrome.[192]

In the intestines, histamine is produced by various cell types, including mast cells in the intestinal mucosa, dendritic cells, and eosinophils.[193] These immune system cell types are a powerful defense mechanism against the bacteria in your gut, providing an essential first line of defense. One of the gastrointestinal disorders in which histamine plays a significant role is Irritable Bowel Syndrome (IBS).

Irritable Bowel Syndrome

Irritable bowel syndrome (IBS) causes abdominal pain, diarrhea, and/or constipation. Researchers believe IBS is a combination of intestinal hypersensitivity along with altered gut bacteria and leaky gut.

---

[192] Deiteren et al., "Histamine H4 Receptors in the Gastrointestinal Tract."
[193] Schirmer and Neumann, "The Function of the Histamine H4 Receptor in Inflammatory and Inflammation-Associated Diseases of the Gut."

The number of mast cells in the intestinal mucosa is elevated in people with IBS, and histamine release in the intestines is part of the IBS symptom cascade. Normally, mast cells make up around 5% of the gut cells in the intestinal barrier area. In addition to having more mast cells in the small intestines, IBS patients have more mast cells located near nerve endings, which may explain the severity of abdominal pain.[194]

In IBS, histamine in the gut is thought to sensitize pain receptors, causing abdominal pain. Mast cells in the gut can be activated by microbes, leading to high histamine levels. The TRPV1 receptor in conjunction with histamine receptor activation sends the signal for pain from neurons in the intestines.[195]

Pro-resolving lipid mediators, such as resolvin 2, are synthesized in the body using omega-3 fatty acids. Researchers have discovered that these mediators may help prevent histamine-induced sensitization of TRPV1 and alleviate pain in IBS.[196] Pro-resolving mediators are synthesized from DHA and EPA, which are omega-3 fatty acids. This makes getting plenty of DHA and EPA a priority for being able to produce resolvins. DHA and EPA are found in marine oils, such as fish oil, krill oil, or algae oil. If you have histamine-related reactions from fish oil, you may want to see if algae oil is a better choice for meeting your DHA and EPA needs.

A low FODMAPs diet is often recommended for people with IBS, and it provides relief for many. Interestingly, a low FODMAPS diet also reduces histamine levels in the intestines. It is thought that lowering the histamine levels by changing the gut microbiome with the low FODMAPs diet decreases the release of histamine from mast cells, breaking the cycle.[197]

---

[194] Hasler et al., "Mast Cell Mediation of Visceral Sensation and Permeability in Irritable Bowel Syndrome."
[195] Hasler et al.
[196] Perna et al., "Effect of Resolvins on Sensitisation of TRPV1 and Visceral Hypersensitivity in IBS."
[197] Uranga, Martínez, and Abalo, "Mast Cell Regulation and Irritable Bowel Syndrome."

A recent study revealed that some IBS patients with high urinary histamine levels also have elevated levels of *Klebsiella aerogenes*, a gut microbe that produces significant amounts of histamine. Reducing fermentable carbohydrates improved symptoms in the study participants, likely by altering the gut microbiome composition. Going deeper into how high histamine in the gut caused pain in IBS patients, the researchers also showed that simply blocking the H4 receptor worked to reduce the IBS symptoms. Additional animal research also clearly showed the role of the histamine H4 receptor in the hypersensitivity to pain in the gut in IBS.[198]

Taken together, the studies show that high histamine levels and activation of histamine receptors may contribute to pain and other symptoms of irritable bowel syndrome.

While histamine contributes to IBS symptoms in the intestines, it can also cause problems in the stomach, such as acid reflux.

Acid Reflux

Whether you call it GERD, heartburn, or acid reflux, high histamine levels can be a cause of excess stomach acid.

There are different causes of heartburn after eating, and you should talk with your doctor if you need help here or have questions.

High histamine levels can cause or exacerbate gastroesophageal reflux disease (GERD). Histamine is released by cells in the stomach in response to food or anticipation of food. The secreted histamine binds to H2 receptors on the type of cells (parietal cells) that release stomach acid, and this triggers the parietal cells to secrete the HCl that makes up stomach acid to break down food. Patients diagnosed with histamine intolerance often have bloating and abdominal pain as symptoms. Some have heartburn and hoarseness as well.[199]

---

[198] De Palma et al., "Histamine Production by the Gut Microbiota Induces Visceral Hyperalgesia through Histamine 4 Receptor Signaling in Mice."
[199] Schnedl et al., "Evaluation of Symptoms and Symptom Combinations in Histamine Intolerance."

If you find that you are reaching for antacids after a meal high in histamine, you may find that DAO enzyme supplements with the meal will help in preventing heartburn. You may also find that reducing the amount of high-histamine foods eaten at dinner may help with preventing acid reflux at night.

In summary, histamine plays a complex role in gastrointestinal disorders such as IBS and acid reflux. By understanding the mechanisms behind histamine's effects on the gut, researchers are discovering new ways to manage these conditions, including dietary changes, enzyme supplements, and targeting specific histamine receptors.

Case Study: The Bloated IT Specialist

Joe is a 33-year-old IT specialist with a main complaint of digestive upset. He started having digestive issues at age 31. He can't really point out a particular event that happened to cause the digestive issues. He has several bowel movements a day that vary from loose to diarrhea and developed hives and itchiness on his skin about 1 hr. after eating. The hives usually go away after a few hours. He also reported having acid reflux when he eats certain foods. He often wakes several times in the middle of the night to go use the bathroom. Several years ago, he did a food sensitivity test, and he avoids the foods that came back as problematic. He continues to have gas and bloating after some meals but not all. He put himself on a gluten free diet assuming that was the cause of his diarrhea. He stopped drinking alcohol 2 years ago because he noticed that it gave him terrible heartburn.

However, despite avoiding the foods that were highlighted as problematic on his food allergy test, he was still having issues.

As a child he had asthma, but he grew out of it. Apart from that, he has had a relatively uneventful life health wise.

He has had multiple tests done to rule out infections in his stomach. He works out daily and leads a fairly easygoing life. He is frustrated because he lacks energy, and he feels terrible in general. He recently saw a practitioner who diagnosed him with SIBO (Small intestinal bacterial overgrowth). He did the SIBO treatment protocol, but his food allergies got worse to the point that eating any kind of protein (animal or plant) caused hives and insomnia.

After doing genomic analysis using a Genetic Lifehacks summary report, it became apparent that Joe had issues with methylation, histamine breakdown in the digestive system and blood stream, low to no *Bifidobacteria*, increased relative risk for wheat allergy and a predisposition to inflammation in the digestive tract.

Supplement Recommendations

- High quality multivitamin with high levels of B12, B6 and B9
- Combination product with Quercetin, Stinging Nettles, NAC, and Bromelain

- Digestive enzymes
- *Bifidobacteria* probiotic

Dietary Recommendations

- Low-histamine diet for 4 weeks
- Food intolerance test for fructose, sorbitol, inulin, and lactose

After 4 weeks, Joe was able to introduce more protein into his diet without having reactions. He was no longer waking up at night to use the bathroom and the incidence of hives and reflux decreased to zero. He also started having more solid stools and less diarrhea. Food intolerance test showed reactions to sorbitol and inulin. It was recommended that he reduce the intake of these foods in his diet.

Chapter 14: Sleep and Circadian Rhythm

Key takeaways:

- In the brain, histamine levels naturally rise in the early morning hours.
- Histamine also plays a role in leg movement during sleep through activation of the H3 receptor.

As a neurotransmitter, histamine's role in brain function is varied. It is involved in wakefulness, mood, neuroinflammation, and even leg movements during sleep. Understanding how high histamine levels affect your sleep and circadian rhythm can help with sleep disorders such as early morning waking. Histamine also plays a role in restless leg and limb movements during sleep.

The Circadian Rhythm of Histamine

Histamine levels naturally ebb and flow in a daily cycle, increasing in the early morning hours and decreasing towards bedtime and overnight. In the brain, histamine acts as a neurotransmitter, promoting alertness and wakefulness. During sleep, adenosine and neurotransmitters like melatonin and serotonin facilitate restfulness. In contrast, histamine, cortisol, and orexin drive wakefulness.

Histamine-related conditions, such as asthma, typically exhibit a circadian bias, with symptom severity worsening between midnight and morning and showing a prominent 24-hour variation.[200]

---

[200] Christ et al., "The Circadian Clock Drives Mast Cell Functions in Allergic Reactions."

The daily fluctuations in histamine levels, with peaks in the early morning and troughs at night, are regulated by the body's circadian rhythm. Circadian rhythm refers to the internal 24-hour clock that governs various physiological processes, including the sleep-wake cycle, hormone production, and metabolism. This internal clock is synchronized with external cues, such as light and darkness, to maintain a consistent daily pattern. The circadian rhythm of histamine is controlled by a set of specific genes that play a crucial role in regulating mast cell activity and histamine release.

Circadian rhythm genes and histamine

Mast cell activity, including baseline histamine release, is governed by circadian rhythm genes. Disruptions in these rhythms, alongside elevated inflammatory cytokines, can lead to increased histamine release in the early morning, potentially causing insomnia.

Circadian rhythm is controlled by a set of core genes, including CLOCK, BMAL1, PER, and CRY. These genes regulate many bodily processes, including histamine release by mast cells. Disruptions in these genes' expression can impact histamine levels and mast cell activity.[201]

Circadian rhythm also impacts how much of a reaction occurs when an allergen binds to the IgE receptor on mast cells. In animal studies, researchers can delete circadian rhythm genes, such as the aptly named CLOCK gene, from the stem cells that generate mast cells. In doing so, researchers have found that the levels of core circadian genes regulate whether an IgE-mediated mast cell degranulation will occur.

Exposure to daylight and the timing of daily activities, such as eating, help reset the circadian rhythm each day. In particular, light in the blue wavelengths plays a crucial role in regulating circadian rhythm genes. Historically, blue light was only available during daylight hours. However, with the advent of modern electric lights, especially LED screens, we are now exposed to blue light at all hours, potentially disrupting our circadian rhythm.

---

[201] Pham et al., "The Interplay between Mast Cells, Pineal Gland, and Circadian Rhythm."

Melatonin is a key hormone in setting your circadian rhythm. The pineal gland releases melatonin in large quantities in the absence of light in the blue wavelengths. Melatonin receptors on mast cells are activated when melatonin levels are high (at night, in the dark). The activation of the melatonin receptor on the surface of the mast cells causes a downregulation within the cell of certain inflammatory molecules, such as NF-kB, which then further decreases the activation and proliferation of mast cells at night.[202] This interaction between melatonin and mast cells is crucial for regulating inflammation and histamine release during the sleep cycle.

While the circadian rhythm of histamine is essential for maintaining a healthy sleep-wake cycle, imbalances in this rhythm can lead to sleep disturbances, such as early morning insomnia

Early Morning Insomnia

Histamine acts as a neurotransmitter in the brain, and it is responsible for wakefulness. Histamine levels rising in the early morning are part of why you feel alert and awake in the morning. Research shows that histamine levels are 3.8 times higher during wakefulness than in sleep in the prefrontal cortex region of the brain.[203] This is a natural response that is part of the daily rhythm and balance of activity.

The most common issue people deal with when histamine levels are too high is waking up around 3 or 4 am with a wide-awake brain. No one enjoys the wide-awake, can't sleep feeling several hours before you normally get up. Your mind may race with worries or thoughts of everything you need to get done for the day. If this happens regularly for you, try tracking whether your early morning waking corresponds to a high histamine meal for dinner. Perhaps you're having an after-dinner dessert containing chocolate – or sipping a cup of cocoa before bed.

Solutions here include:

- Eating a low-histamine meal for dinner

---

[202] Pham et al.

[203] Chu et al., "Extracellular Histamine Level in the Frontal Cortex Is Positively Correlated with the Amount of Wakefulness in Rats."

- Taking a DAO enzyme supplement with dinner or dessert
- Get your circadian rhythm back on track
  - Try a week with no electronics (blue light emitting screens) for two hours before bedtime
  - Get out in the sun for daylight exposure in the morning

Try tracking these interventions and see if your sleep improves after a couple of nights. You might be surprised by the positive impact these simple changes can have on your sleep quality.

In addition to its role in early morning insomnia, histamine has also been implicated in other sleep disorders, such as periodic limb movement disorder (PLMD) and restless leg syndrome (RLS).

Periodic Limb Movement in Sleep and Restless Leg Syndrome

Research also points to histamine and histamine receptors being involved in sleep disorders, such as periodic limb movement disorder (PLMD) or restless leg syndrome (RLS).

Periodic limb movement disorder (PLMD) is a sleep disorder in which the legs, feet, arms, or hands rhythmically move during sleep. This could be a rhythmic leg jerk that happens periodically in 30-second intervals or a rhythmic hand tapping. The standard of care for PLMD is Parkinson's medications, which only work for a percentage of people with PLMD.

A 2020 study in animals found that the H3 histamine receptor in the brain is likely involved in PLMD. Blocking the H3 receptor with an experimental drug stopped leg movement in sleep. Additionally, brain samples in the animals with PLMD showed much higher H3 receptor levels in the striatum, which is the region that controls motor activity.[204]

---

[204] Lai et al., "Striatal Histamine Mechanism in the Pathogenesis of Restless Legs Syndrome."

The H3 receptor in the brain regulates histamine release by negative feedback. The H3 receptor also regulates the release of dopamine, GABA, and acetylcholine in certain areas of the brain. The H3 receptor is an area of ongoing research as a drug target for psychiatric disorders and sleep disorders. Currently, an H3 receptor inverse agonist, pitolisant, is approved for treating narcolepsy.[205]

There is an overlap with PLMD being found in many people with restless leg syndrome, although it can be found as a separate condition for some people. A study involving patients with mast cell activation syndrome found that they were about 3 times more likely to have restless leg syndrome than a control group.[206]

The research on histamine and striatal histamine receptors in PLMD and RLS is relatively new and not yet conclusive, suggesting that multiple pathways may be involved. However, if you are experiencing other high histamine symptoms alongside PLMD or RLS, addressing histamine imbalances may be the key to relief.

In conclusion, histamine plays a vital role in regulating sleep and circadian rhythm. The natural ebb and flow of histamine levels throughout the day, governed by circadian rhythm genes, is essential for maintaining a healthy sleep-wake cycle. Disruptions in this balance can lead to various sleep disturbances, such as early morning insomnia, periodic limb movement disorder, and restless leg syndrome. Importantly, melatonin helps to tamp down mast cell activation at night. Decreasing your exposure to blue light in the evening may help to reduce your overall histamine load, providing health benefits into the next day.

---

[205] Peng et al., "Structural Basis for Recognition of Antihistamine Drug by Human Histamine Receptor."
[206] Weinstock et al., "Restless Legs Syndrome Is Associated with Mast Cell Activation Syndrome."

Case Study: Sleep, Anxiety, and Gut Issues

Sandra is a 65-year-old menopausal woman with a lifelong history of digestive issues. Over the years, she has seen different practitioners and tried different treatments however her symptoms never seem to resolve for good. She remembered being told by her mother that she was a colicky baby. She identified as being a somewhat anxious person who worries a lot about everything.

Her main symptoms were lots of gas and occasional intermittent bloating. She described her abdomen as feeling tight like a drum and it can be very painful. She experiences mostly constipation but has had diarrhea on a few occasions.

In addition, she suffers from insomnia (difficulties falling and staying asleep), heartburn and itchy skin that comes and goes. She often experiences food reactions up to 3 days after eating. This has made it difficult to know what is causing her digestive issues.

She maintains a gluten and dairy-free diet, and this has helped a little bit but not completely. She noticed that alcohol in particular red wine makes her heartburn much worse. The only time she had complete relief from her symptoms was when she tried a very restrictive Low FODMAP diet for 1 year; however, she stopped because it was too difficult to maintain the restrictive diet.

Treatment for histamine intolerance is often multifaceted and multimodal.

Supplement recommendations:

- Quercetin dihydrate + vitamin C were recommended for mast cell stabilization
- Vitamin D - stabilize mast cells and decrease inflammation
- Histamine DAO - degrades histamine in the digestive tract
- *Bacillus coagulans,* a spore based probiotic
- L-theanine + GABA combination at bedtime to decrease mast cell activation and promote relaxation

Dietary Recommendations

- Low FODMAP diet was recommended for 3 months
- Herbal antimicrobial with oil of oregano, allicin, and coptis

Lifestyle Recommendations

- Gut hypnosis for stress management - 1-3 times per day depending on stress levels
- Circadian rhythm reset: bright light for 30 mins in the morning with elimination of blue light at night.

Three months into the program, Sandra was doing much better and able to start introducing moderate histamine foods into her diet. She discovered that wine in particular causes all her previous symptoms to recur, but a serving of tequila or gin does not cause any health issues.

Chapter 15: Estrogen, Histamine, and Mast Cell Interaction: A Complex Interplay

Key takeaways:

- Mast cells, which release histamine, may be more easily triggered when estrogen levels are high.
- Histamine in foods contributes to overall histamine levels in the body.
- Genetic variants affect the breakdown and elimination of histamine.
- Endocrine disruptors like BPA and PFOAs can activate estrogen receptors on mast cells, increasing histamine release.

Estrogen plays a complex role in the body's histamine response, particularly regarding mast cell activation. Both men and women produce estrogen, but its levels and effects vary by sex and age. This chapter dives into the interplay between estrogen, histamine intolerance, and mast cell activation, shedding light on how these factors contribute to health and well-being.

Estrogen and Mast Cell Activation

Estrogen operates by binding to estrogen receptors (ERα, ERβ, and GPER1) in various tissues, including the heart, brain, muscles, and immune system. It can initiate gene transcription and immediate cellular responses. Estradiol (E2) is the primary active form of estrogen produced before menopause.

Research indicates that high levels of estradiol can prompt mast cells to release histamine. Fluctuations in estrogen levels, particularly in women, may heighten sensitivity to mast cell activation, potentially explaining the prevalence of certain symptoms in women, especially during periods of hormonal change like perimenopause.[207]

However, research indicates that consistently elevated estrogen levels, as observed in estrogen dominance, can lead to the downregulation of estrogen receptors on mast cells. Consequently, fluctuations in estrogen levels or exposure to excess estrogen may be problematic for individuals with easily activated mast cells.[208]

Estrogen plays a role in mast cell-mediated diseases, such as allergies and asthma. While boys are more likely to have asthma in childhood, that ratio switches in young adults. Asthma and other allergic diseases of the airway are about three times more common in women than men during their reproductive years when estrogen levels are higher. Asthma symptoms worsen in many women during the high-estrogen phase right before their period. In addition, asthma rates are higher in post-menopausal women who are taking hormone replacement therapy.[209]

In addition to the effects of endogenous estrogen on mast cells, environmental compounds that mimic estrogen can also influence mast cell activation.

Environmental estrogen-mimics

Compounds like BPA and PFOAs, found in plastics and other consumer products, can mimic estrogen, and bind to its receptors, including the estrogen receptors on mast cells. Animal research shows that the interaction with environmental estrogens can amplify the effects of estrogen in the body and increase mast cell activation with histamine release.[210]

---

[207] Zaitsu et al., "Estradiol Activates Mast Cells via a Non-Genomic Estrogen Receptor-α and Calcium Influx."

[208] Nesheim et al., "Elevated Seminal Plasma Estradiol and Epigenetic Inactivation of ESR1 and ESR2 Is Associated with CP/CPPS."

[209] Zierau, Zenclussen, and Jensen, "Role of Female Sex Hormones, Estradiol and Progesterone, in Mast Cell Behavior."

[210] O'Brien, Dolinoy, and Mancuso, "Perinatal Bisphenol A Exposures Increase Production of Pro-Inflammatory Mediators in Bone Marrow-Derived Mast Cells of Adult Mice."

While estrogen and environmental estrogens can impact mast cell activation peripherally, estrogen also interacts with histamine in the brain.

Estrogen and Histamine in the Brain

Histamine as a neurotransmitter in the brain can have both excitatory and inhibitory effects, depending on the type of receptor to which it binds and the cell type. The number of histamine receptors on the surface of neurons can impact the action that happens with the cell.

Importantly, estrogen influences the expression of histamine receptors in the brain. An animal study demonstrated that estrogen stimulation influenced the level of H1 receptors in the hypothalamus.[211] Furthermore, estrogen can also modulate histamine levels in the brain, which affects appetite control. Researchers think that this potentially contributes to weight gain during menopause.[212]

The interplay between estrogen and histamine extends beyond the brain and is particularly relevant during pregnancy, a period characterized by significant hormonal changes.

Pregnancy and Histamine:

During pregnancy, the body undergoes significant changes in immune function and hormone levels, which can affect histamine balance. Many women report that their allergies and food intolerances improve during pregnancy, and this may be due to the increased production of diamine oxidase (DAO) by the placenta.

[211] Mori et al., "Estrogenic Regulation of Histamine Receptor Subtype H1 Expression in the Ventromedial Nucleus of the Hypothalamus in Female Rats."
[212] Gotoh et al., "Hypothalamic Neuronal Histamine Signaling in the Estrogen Deficiency-Induced Obesity."

DAO is the primary enzyme responsible for breaking down histamine in the body. The placenta produces a large amount of DAO, which helps to regulate histamine levels during pregnancy. This increased DAO production may contribute to the alleviation of histamine-related symptoms in pregnant women. The balance of histamine and DAO is important in pregnancy, and reduced DAO levels are found in pregnancy disorders, such as premature rupture of membranes and pre-eclampsia.

Histamine is thought to be important during the implantation period, and histamine levels during the first month or two of pregnancy remain higher. To protect the fetus from the potential harm of excessive histamine, DAO production increases significantly in the second and third trimesters, leading to a significant decline in maternal blood histamine levels.[213] Animal studies clearly show that high histamine levels are detrimental to the fetus in the later stages of pregnancy, so DAO production increases to protect the fetus from too much histamine.[214]

To illustrate the complex interactions between estrogen, histamine, and mast cells, let's consider the case of Callie, a perimenopausal CEO struggling with various health concerns.

---

[213] Brew and Sullivan, "The Links between Maternal Histamine Levels and Complications of Human Pregnancy."
[214] Maintz et al., "Effects of Histamine and Diamine Oxidase Activities on Pregnancy."

Case Study: Perimenopausal CEO

Callie was a lovely 44-year-old CEO for a tech startup company. She initially came to me for irregular menstrual cycles, weight gain and digestive disturbance. She has a long-standing history of constipation and digestive ailments that come and go. Currently she has been experiencing mainly bloating and constipation. She has also noticed that her sleep is off, and she often has a difficult time falling asleep due to a busy mind. She gets up one to two times in the middle of the night to use the washroom.

Other health concerns were rashes on her arms and stomach, difficulties losing fat around her abdomen and migraines especially close to her menses.

She became aware that whenever she drinks alcohol, she is completely wiped out and unable to function for the next two days. She also started having more migraines around her menstrual cycle.

Callie agreed to do dried urine hormone testing. She also did genetic testing. Three months into the hormone rebalancing protocol she mentioned that her symptoms have not gotten significantly better, and her digestive concerns seem to be worsening.

A Genetic Lifehacks summary report was generated, and it was discovered that Callie had genetic variants that affected the methylation and histaminergic pathways. She was not clearing out histamine effectively from the digestive tract and systemically. In addition, her Phase II detoxification pathways were not efficient. A slow Phase II detoxification and methylation pathway can lead to an increased estrogen load in the body.

Dietary Recommendations

- Increase intake of cruciferous vegetables to help with Phase II detoxification
- Low FODMAP x 4 weeks to calm down the digestive tract and encourage better bowel movements
- Meal spacing technique for sluggish bowels: eat 3 meals a day spaced 4-5 hours apart. No snacks during the day. The last meal of the day must be eaten at least 3 hours before bed

- Do a 12 hour overnight fast to regulate the Migrating Motor Complex
- Avoid fermented foods and histamine liberators and alcohol

Supplement Recommendations

- High-quality multivitamin to support the methylation cycle
- Magnesium glycinate - support methylation, detoxification of estrogen and improves sleep
- Combination product with DIM, indole 3 carbinol, sulforaphane glucosinolate, calcium D-glucarate, milk thistle, alpha lipoic acid, and N-acetyl L-cysteine - helps to support estrogen metabolism and liver detoxification
- Vitex - supports progesterone levels in the body
- Hist DAO - helps to breakdown histamine in the digestive tract

Lifestyle Recommendations

- Mindfulness meditation 15 minutes in the morning and 15 minutes in the evening
- Journaling for 10 minutes each night to calm the mind
- Gentle walking in the evenings after dinner for 30 mins
- Increase yoga practice from once a week to two times a week for stress management

It was recommended to Callie to get breath testing for Small Intestinal Bacterial Overgrowth (SIBO) as a reason her digestive concerns are not resolving permanently.

Chapter 16: Histamine, Asthma, and the Lungs

Key takeaways:

- Histamine release is part of the bronchoconstriction in asthma and airway hypersensitivity.
- Mast cell activation and the release of histamine plays a role in asthma attacks.

Mast cells line the lungs, playing a crucial role in the body's defense against inhaled pathogens such as viruses and bacteria. Asthma has been linked to inappropriate mast cell activation and histamine release for decades. However, recent discoveries have provided a more comprehensive understanding of this relationship.

When histamine is released in the lungs, it contributes to airway sensitivity and asthma in three ways:[215]

- **Bronchoconstriction:** Histamine causes smooth muscle contractions around the airways (bronchoconstriction), leading to the narrowing of the airways.
- **Increased Mucus Production:** It stimulates the mucus glands in the airways, leading to increased production of mucus, which can further block airways.
- **Inflammation and Swelling:** Histamine contributes to inflammation and swelling in the airways, exacerbating the narrowing and obstruction caused by smooth muscle contraction.

These actions are mainly due to the activation of H1 receptors in the lungs. While these are all roles of histamine elsewhere in the body, when it happens in the lungs, it can be particularly harmful.

---

[215] Yamauchi and Ogasawara, "The Role of Histamine in the Pathophysiology of Asthma and the Clinical Efficacy of Antihistamines in Asthma Therapy."

Asthma: Histamine Causes Bronchoconstriction

Asthma can be classified into two main types: allergic asthma and non-allergic asthma. Allergic asthma is triggered by IgE-mediated allergen activation of the airways, while non-allergic asthma does not involve traditional allergens

For both triggers of asthma, the accumulation of mast cells in the lungs is key. While mast cells are present in everyone's lungs as part of the innate immune response, studies have demonstrated an increased number of lung mast cells in individuals with asthma. Furthermore, the repeated release of histamine activates H4 receptors on mast cells, promoting the recruitment of additional mast cells to the affected area of the lungs.[216] [217]

Mast cells can be activated by various particles that bind to toll-like receptors (TLRs) on the cell surface, such as TLR-1 and TLR-4. These receptors respond to lipopolysaccharides from gram-negative bacteria, as well as fungal species and mycotoxins from mold. In addition, allergens can trigger mast cells in the lungs through IgE-mediated activation. All of these mechanisms can contribute to the activation of asthma

Genetic studies also highlight the important role of histamine in airway hypersensitivity. Histamine N-methyltransferase (HNMT), the primary enzyme responsible for breaking down and eliminating histamine in the airways, has been implicated in asthma risk. Genetic variants in the HNMT gene and the H1 receptor gene have been associated with an increased susceptibility to asthma.[218]

While both allergic and non-allergic asthma involve mast cell activation and histamine release, the underlying mechanisms differ. Let's look at both types in more detail:

---

[216] Banafea et al., "The Role of Human Mast Cells in Allergy and Asthma."

[217] Méndez-Enríquez and Hallgren, "Mast Cells and Their Progenitors in Allergic Asthma."

[218] Yamauchi and Ogasawara, "The Role of Histamine in the Pathophysiology of Asthma and the Clinical Efficacy of Antihistamines in Asthma Therapy."

Non-allergic asthma

Non-allergic asthma is more common in adults, while allergic asthma is the most common type in children. IgE-independent activation of mast cells plays a role in non-allergic asthma.

Individuals with long-term, chronic asthma often experience changes in their airways, a process known as airway remodeling. This remodeling is thought to be caused by the release of tryptase and histamine from mast cells, leading to an increase in type I collagen formation. Chronic inflammation can result in long-term alterations in the airways, making them more sensitive and reactive to triggers.[219]

In asthma, mast cells can be activated by cold air or by exercise, in addition to particles that are inhaled or viral infections. Recent research has implicated the MRGPRX2 receptor on mast cells in non-allergic asthma. A study found that MRGPRX2 expression is elevated in the lungs of individuals with asthma compared to those without the condition. The activation of MRGPRX2 receptors in asthma may be triggered by various factors, including viral respiratory infections, substance P, or certain types of drugs.[220]

In contrast to non-allergic asthma, allergic asthma is characterized by IgE-mediated mast cell activation in response to specific allergens.

Allergic asthma

In allergic asthma, the activation of mast cells and release of histamine and tryptase are triggered by IgE stimulation from an allergen.

For example, in someone who is allergic to dust mites, particles from dust mites in the air can activate the IgE receptors on cells in the lungs. This triggers immediate mast cell degranulation, and the flood of histamine causes bronchoconstriction, swelling, and mucus production. Studies on histamine in asthma show that certain H1 receptor blockers help to reduce histamine and decrease the bronchoconstriction from allergens.

---

[219] Komi et al., "The Role of Mast Cells in IgE-Independent Lung Diseases."
[220] Méndez-Enríquez and Hallgren, "Mast Cells and Their Progenitors in Allergic Asthma."

Chapter 17: Bladder and Prostate Problems

Key takeaways:

- Mast cells are abundant in the bladder and prostate, and their activation can contribute to various urological problems.

- Elevated histamine levels and mast cell activation play a significant role in the development of interstitial cystitis.

- Prostate enlargement, such as benign prostatic hyperplasia (BPH), can also involve histamine and mast cell activation as a component of the disease process.

Mast cells are also abundant in the bladder and the prostate, leading to problems when mast cells are activated there. The bladder lining and the muscles responsible for bladder contractions contain all four histamine receptors: H1, H2, H3, and H4.[221]

Interstitial Cystitis:

Interstitial cystitis (IC) is a condition in which the bladder wall can become irritated and cause the bladder to feel more sensitive than normal. Essentially, it feels like a bladder infection, but without the infection. Painful bladder syndrome is another term.

Elevated histamine levels and mast cell activation can be a contributing factor in interstitial cystitis.[222] Be sure to talk with your doctor, though, if you have questions about bladder symptoms, as there may be multiple causes that require further investigation.

---

[221] Stromberga, Chess-Williams, and Moro, "Histamine Modulation of Urinary Bladder Urothelium, Lamina Propria and Detrusor Contractile Activity via H1 and H2 Receptors."
[222] Malik et al., "Distribution of Mast Cell Subtypes in Interstitial Cystitis."

Mast cells line the bladder and can be activated by pathogens or environmental toxins. They are an important part of the innate immune response in the bladder. However, mast cell release of histamine and other mediators can cause the irritation, pain, and urgency that is associated with a bladder infection - but without the infection.

Have you ever noticed that your bladder symptoms worsen during periods of stress? This could be due to high histamine levels resulting from mast cell activation in the bladder. Animal studies have demonstrated that stress can activate mast cells in the bladder. In one study, psychological stress was found to trigger approximately 70% of the mast cells lining the bladder.[223]

I want to be clear here: Histamine and mast cell activation likely aren't the sole cause of interstitial cystitis symptoms. Other receptors and nerve activation are also involved in IC. However, if you have IC plus other histamine-related symptoms, you may find that your IC symptoms improve when lowering overall histamine levels.

In addition to interstitial cystitis, mast cell activation, and histamine release may also play a role in another common urological condition: overactive bladder.

Overactive Bladder

An overactive bladder causes the feeling of needing to urgently head to the bathroom. The urge to urinate may be hard to control, and incontinence is frequently a problem for people with overactive bladder. In addition, needing to get up in the night to go to the bathroom can interfere with sleep quality.

[223] Spanos et al., "Stress-Induced Bladder Mast Cell Activation."

People with overactive bladder have more mast cells in the lining of their bladders than normal. A study involving bladder wall biopsies in patients with overactive bladder and interstitial cystitis compared to a control group showed that mast cell numbers were more than doubled in the bladder lining for both interstitial cystitis and overactive bladder. It's also important to know what isn't involved in the bladder issues. The study ruled out differences in cell-to-cell adhesion molecules as a cause of overactive bladder. [224]

Histamine in the Prostate

Prostate problems, such as benign prostate hyperplasia (BPH), are common in older men and often coexist with lower urinary tract symptoms. This combination can significantly impact the quality of life for many individuals. Animal studies clearly show that prostate inflammation, fibrosis, and urinary dysfunction involve mast cell activation, histamine release, and histamine receptor activations.

To illustrate this point, let's look at a couple of studies:

When looking at the receptors involved in BPH, one study found that a mast cell inhibitor, cromolyn sodium, combined with an H1 receptor blocker, cetirizine, reduced urinary issues as well as reduced fibrosis in the prostate.[225]

A study in men with BPH demonstrated that chronic activation of inflammatory pathways, such as from bacterial antigens, chemical irritants, and other causes of inflammation, causes hyperproliferation in benign prostate hyperplasia. The study showed that the inflammatory cell types included T lymphocytes, macrophages, and mast cells.[226] Thus, mast cells play a role in prostate problems, but similarly to the studies on interstitial cystitis, the histamine release from mast cells is only part of the picture.

---

[224] Liu et al., "Differences in Mast Cell Infiltration, E-Cadherin, and Zonula Occludens-1 Expression Between Patients With Overactive Bladder and Interstitial Cystitis/Bladder Pain Syndrome."
[225] Pattabiraman et al., "Mast Cell Function in Prostate Inflammation, Fibrosis, and Smooth Muscle Cell Dysfunction."
[226] Krušlin et al., "Inflammation in Prostatic Hyperplasia and Carcinoma—Basic Scientific Approach."

Research also shows that both histamine and the H3 receptor are overexpressed in prostate cancer cells. Studies in animals show that blocking the H3 receptor, which can act as a negative feedback loop in some cell types, significantly inhibits prostate tumor growth.[227] Keep in mind that these are just animal and cell line studies and that blocking the H3 receptor needs to be tested in men with prostate cancer to know if it is effective.

The complex interplay between histamine, mast cell activation, and urological disorders is exemplified in the case of Jamila, a university professor struggling with irritable bladder and digestive issues. Her story demonstrates how addressing underlying factors such as SIBO, histamine intolerance, and stress management can lead to improvements in bladder symptoms and overall quality of life.

---

[227] Chen and Hu, "Inhibition of Histamine Receptor H3R Suppresses Prostate Cancer Growth, Invasion and Increases Apoptosis via the AR Pathway."

Case Study: The Overactive Professor

Jamila is a 38-year-old university professor who presented with chief symptoms of digestive upset and irritable bladder. She complained of excessive bloating and gas with abdominal cramps no matter what she ate. She noticed that she would often have multiple bowel movements in a day. Her complaints of bladder pain, lower abdominal pain, urgency and frequency really started to get worse 2 years before she met me. In addition, she was extremely fatigued with brain fog and weight gain. All in all, Jamila was not a happy woman.

During our initial appointment, I noticed that Jamila was very talkative with a typical Type A personality profile. Although she loved her job, she was under quite a bit of stress, and she didn't really have a lot of outlets to relax and recharge.

She was very accomplished in her career. As the assistant dean of her department at her university, she liked to research everything and had lots of questions. Her health was very important to her and by the time I saw her, she had already seen a few other practitioners and done a ton of research into her health issues. She was on a lot of supplements (fourteen to be exact) and had been trying different things with her diet for the past 2 years.

In addition to having an irritable bladder and digestive issues, she was also dealing with seasonal allergies, painful heavy menses, pain with intercourse and acne breakouts that were affecting her self-esteem.

Due to her extensive digestive issues, a SIBO breath test was done to see if it was a contributing factor to her health complaints. Her breath test did come back positive for SIBO (Small Intestinal Bacterial Overgrowth). She agreed to treat her digestive concerns to see if it would settle her acne breakouts and bladder issues.

After undergoing SIBO eradication treatment, she noticed that her bladder symptoms improved but did not completely resolve. At least she wasn't in excruciating pain anymore and she was having less bloating and gas.

After careful examination of Jamila's genomics, she had SNPs for cortisol regulation/stress response, methylation, inflammation, and decreased histamine clearance from the digestive tract and systemically.

It was decided that the focus would shift to addressing histamine intolerance since Jamila had a reduction in bladder symptoms by addressing SIBO and doing a Low FODMAP diet. There is research to show that a Low FODMAP diet is helpful in individuals with histamine intolerance. We also decided that Jamila's high stress job and personality was probably contributing to her bladder irritability and digestive complaints.

By focusing on histamine intolerance and stress management techniques, Jamila was able to calm the inflammation in her body and work toward a better quality of life.

Supplement Recommendation

- Combination product containing: Berberine, thyme, cinnamon, neem, uva ursi, and oregano extracts - used for eradication of intestinal microbes in SIBO
- Quercetin - stabilizes mast cells
- Hesperidin - reduces histamine release and number of H1 receptors available for histamine to bind to
- Nonirritating option for people with sensitive bladders
- Bioactive curcumin - anti-inflammatory and uroprotective
- L glutamine - decreases inflammatory response in the bladder and intestines, supports the microbiome, and improves bladder and gut lining

Dietary Recommendations

- Low FODMAP diet x 12 weeks to eradicate SIBO
- Limit bladder irritating foods such as: chocolate, tomatoes, lemon/limes, vinegars, spicy foods, apples, peaches, strawberries, cranberries, black and green tea, and coffee.
- Keep a diet diary as moderate to higher FODMAPs are brought back into the diet to figure out hidden triggers

Lifestyle Recommendations

- Mindfulness walking meditation - 10 mins at least 3 times a week

- Walking in nature 2-3 times a week to regulate the autonomic nervous system
- Reading/journaling in the evenings to calm down the nervous system
- Encouraged Jamila to start to engage in a hobby/activity that brings her joy

Chapter 18: Concluding Thoughts

Throughout this book, we've explored the complex role of histamine in the body and how imbalances can lead to a wide range of health issues. From understanding the biochemistry of histamine creation and its interactions with various receptors to recognizing the impact of mast cell activation on multiple body systems, we've covered a lot of ground. We've also delved into the genetic factors that influence histamine balance, the role of the gut microbiome, and the importance of dietary and lifestyle modifications in managing histamine-related symptoms.

I wanted to wrap up with what I think are the most important points to remember:

High histamine levels can affect many different systems in the body and lowering histamine levels can help to down-regulate histamine receptors and get you off the histamine merry-go-round.

Genetic variants can play a role in susceptibility to histamine issues, but they aren't usually the sole cause. Instead, genetics may tip one person over the edge into histamine issues, while another person can handle the load.

A low-histamine diet can be a great tool for resetting your histamine levels and lowering your overall histamine burden. The goal with a low-histamine diet is to use it as a temporary reset, and then gradually add back in many of the health foods that contain histamine.

The gut microbiome is an often-overlooked source of histamine in the body. From dietary changes to encouraging good gut bacteria to choosing the right probiotics (and avoiding the wrong ones), your gut microbiome can help you overcome high histamine symptoms.

It is important to address histamine-related health issues from a holistic perspective. There is no one-size-fits-all solution, and the most effective approach often involves a combination of strategies tailored to your unique needs and circumstances.

While it can often be frustrating to find the right doctor or healthcare professional, I want to encourage you to seek professional help as needed. Having a strong healthcare ally in your corner can make a big difference in finding the right solutions for you.

As we conclude, I want to remind you that you have the power to make positive changes in your life.

Appendix:

Low-histamine diet foods list:

This list was adapted from several sources including the Swiss Interest Group Histamine Intolerance. It is based on many sources, including reported food intolerances by patients. You may find that some foods on this list don't bother you.

Eggs and dairy products high in histamine:

- Blue cheese
- Cheddar cheese
- Mature, hard cheeses (e.g., parmesan)
- Fontina cheese
- Gouda, mature
- Raw milk cheeses
- Rochefort cheese
- Egg whites, raw

Meat, fish, and seafood:

- Dried meats (e.g., beef jerky)
- Ham
- Salami
- Sausages
- Smoked fish
- Smoked meat
- Anchovies
- Any fish or seafood that isn't fresh
- Crab
- Bivalves
- Crawfish
- Lobster
- Shrimp

Grains:

- Barley
- Buckwheat

Nuts:

- Pecans
- Walnuts

Vegetables:

- Avocado
- Chickpeas
- Eggplant
- Hot peppers
- Kelp (brown seaweeds)
- Lentils
- Olives
- Pickled vegetables
- Pulses
- Sauerkraut
- Spinach
- Stinging nettle
- Soybeans
- Tomato

Fruits:

- Citrus fruits (may liberate histamine for some people)
- Papaya
- Pineapple
- Raspberry
- Strawberry

Spices, seasoning:

- Cumin
- Chocolate
- Curry

- Licorice root
- Mustard seed
- Paprika, hot
- Pepper
- Soy Sauce
- Vinegars

Beverages:

- Black tea
- Chocolate drinks
- Soy milk
- Tomato juice
- Beverages that contain alcohol

Additives and food coloring:

- Many preservatives and food colorings seem to trigger histamine release in people who are sensitive to high-histamine foods.

Prescription drugs that interact with histamine:

Please talk with your doctor about any questions you have about medications before stopping a prescription.

Adapted from
https://www.ncbi.nlm.nih.gov/pmc/articles/PMC8308327/table/nutrients-13-02228-t002/

Prescription drugs interfering with histamine metabolism or distribution

Prokinetics:	metoclopramide
Antiinfectives:	clavulanic acid, isoniazid, cefuroxime, cefotiame, pentamidine, chloroquine, doxycycline, neomycin B, acriflavine, D-cycloserine
Bronchodilators:	aminophylline, theophylline
Diuretics:	amiloride, furosemide
Antidepressants:	amitriptyline, monoaminooxidase 1 inhibitors
Anxiolytics:	diazepam, barbiturates
Antipsychotics:	haloperidol
Cytostatics:	cyclophosphamide
Antihypertensives:	verapamil, dihydrazine, alprenolol
Cardiotonics:	dobutamine, dopamine
Opioids:	pethidine, morphine, codeine
Analgesics:	metamizole
Local anaesthetics:	lidocaine, prilocaine, marcaine, procaine
General anaesthetics:	thiopental
Muscle relaxants:	pancuronium, alcuronium, D-tubocurarine
Antiarrhytmics:	propafenone, verapamil, quinidine
Radiocontrast agents:	iodine containing

Meal ideas:

Stuck on where to start with a low-histamine diet? Here are several meal ideas to get you started.

Breakfast Ideas:

Oatmeal with fresh apples and a drizzle of maple syrup

1. Cook old-fashioned oats in water or milk (if tolerated)
2. Top with sliced fresh apples
3. Drizzle with a small amount of maple syrup for sweetness

Quinoa breakfast bowl with peaches and pumpkin seeds

1. Cook quinoa in water or milk (if tolerated) according to package instructions
2. Top with fresh peach slices and a handful of pumpkin seeds
3. Optional: add a splash of vanilla extract for flavor

Scrambled eggs with sautéed kale and sweet potatoes

1. Sauté fresh kale in a pan with a little olive oil until wilted
2. Scramble eggs in a separate pan
3. Serve eggs and spinach with roasted or boiled sweet potato slices
4. Optional: add salt and pepper (if it doesn't bother you) to taste

Overnight oats with blueberries and chia seeds

1. Mix old-fashioned oats, milk (if tolerated), and a little honey in a jar or bowl
2. Add fresh or frozen blueberries and a tablespoon of chia seeds
3. Let sit overnight in the refrigerator
4. In the morning, give the oats a stir and add a splash of milk if needed to achieve desired consistency

Lunch ideas:

Quinoa and vegetable salad

1. Cook quinoa according to package instructions and let cool
2. Mix cooled quinoa with diced cucumber, grated carrots, and chopped bell peppers
3. Dress with a simple olive oil and lemon juice dressing
4. Optional: add fresh herbs like basil or parsley for flavor

Grilled chicken breast with roasted Brussels sprouts and sweet potatoes

1. Season chicken breast with salt, pepper, and garlic powder, then grill until cooked through
2. Toss Brussels sprouts and sweet potato wedges with olive oil, salt, and pepper, then roast in the oven until tender
3. Serve grilled chicken alongside roasted vegetables

Turkey and cucumber wraps

1. Spread a thin layer of hummus on a wrap or lettuce leaf
2. Layer with sliced turkey breast, cucumber slices, and fresh sprouts or microgreens
3. Roll up the wrap and slice it in half
4. Optional: add a side of carrot and celery sticks for crunch

Dinner Ideas:

Baked salmon with asparagus and brown rice

1. Season fresh salmon fillets with salt, pepper, and lemon juice, then bake in the oven until cooked through. If very fresh salmon isn't available, use frozen salmon that is quickly thawed in a bowl of cold water. Look for "frozen at sea" with fish or seafood.
2. Steam or sauté asparagus spears until tender-crisp
3. Serve salmon and asparagus over cooked brown rice
4. Optional: garnish with fresh dill or parsley

Turkey and vegetable stir-fry

1. Stir-fry sliced turkey breast, broccoli florets, sliced bell peppers, and sliced zucchini in a pan with olive oil
2. Season with salt, pepper, and a very small amount of low-sodium soy sauce or coconut aminos (if they don't bother you)
3. Serve over cooked quinoa or rice

Lamb and vegetable curry

1. Sauté diced onions, garlic, and ginger in a pot with olive oil until softened
2. Add diced lamb, low-sodium vegetable broth, and diced sweet potatoes, carrots, and cauliflower florets to the pot
3. Simmer until lamb and vegetables are tender
4. Season with salt, pepper (if it doesn't bother you), and mild curry powder (without chili)
5. Serve over cooked basmati rice

Pizza:

1. Create a fresh pizza dough or use pizza dough from the deli at your grocery store
2. Avoid the tomato sauce. Instead, try Alfredo sauce or olive oil and garlic
3. Top with fresh mozzarella, fresh basil, roasted red peppers, freshly cooked chicken breast, onions, zucchini, and artichoke hearts (in oil, not vinegar)

References

Adams, Karla E., and Tonya S. Rans. "Adverse Reactions to Alcohol and Alcoholic Beverages." *Annals of Allergy, Asthma & Immunology* 111, no. 6 (December 1, 2013): 439–45. https://doi.org/10.1016/j.anai.2013.09.016.

Al Bulushi, Ismail, Susan Poole, Hilton C. Deeth, and Gary A. Dykes. "Biogenic Amines in Fish: Roles in Intoxication, Spoilage, and Nitrosamine Formation--a Review." *Critical Reviews in Food Science and Nutrition* 49, no. 4 (April 2009): 369–77. https://doi.org/10.1080/10408390802067514.

Arriaga-Gomez, Erica, Jaclyn Kline, Elizabeth Emanuel, Nefeli Neamonitaki, Tenzin Yangdon, Hayley Zacheis, Dogukan Pasha, et al. "Repeated Vaginal Exposures to the Common Cosmetic and Household Preservative Methylisothiazolinone Induce Persistent, Mast Cell-Dependent Genital Pain in ND4 Mice." *International Journal of Molecular Sciences* 20, no. 21 (October 28, 2019): 5361. https://doi.org/10.3390/ijms20215361.

Averina, Maria, Jan Brox, Sandra Huber, Anne-Sofie Furberg, and Martin Sørensen. "Serum Perfluoroalkyl Substances (PFAS) and Risk of Asthma and Various Allergies in Adolescents. The Tromsø Study Fit Futures in Northern Norway." *Environmental Research* 169 (February 1, 2019): 114–21. https://doi.org/10.1016/j.envres.2018.11.005.

Ayudhya, Chalatip Chompunud Na, and Hydar Ali. "MRGPRX2 and Its Role in Non-IgE-Mediated Drug Hypersensitivity." *Immunology and Allergy Clinics of North America* 42, no. 2 (May 2022): 269–84. https://doi.org/10.1016/j.iac.2021.12.003.

Ayuso, Pedro, Elena García-Martín, Carmen Martínez, and José A. G. Agúndez. "Genetic Variability of Human Diamine Oxidase: Occurrence of Three Nonsynonymous Polymorphisms and Study of Their Effect on Serum Enzyme Activity."

Pharmacogenetics and Genomics 17, no. 9 (September 2007): 687–93. https://doi.org/10.1097/FPC.0b013e328012b8e4.

Banafea, Ghalya H, Sherin Bakhashab, Huda F Alshaibi, Peter Natesan Pushparaj, and Mahmood Rasool. "The Role of Human Mast Cells in Allergy and Asthma." *Bioengineered* 13, no. 3 (n.d.): 7049–64. https://doi.org/10.1080/21655979.2022.2044278.

Bilotta, Sabrina, Lakshmi Bhargavi Paruchuru, Katharina Feilhauer, Jörg Köninger, and Axel Lorentz. "Resveratrol Is a Natural Inhibitor of Human Intestinal Mast Cell Activation and Phosphorylation of Mitochondrial ERK1/2 and STAT3." *International Journal of Molecular Sciences* 22, no. 14 (July 16, 2021): 7640. https://doi.org/10.3390/ijms22147640.

Bover-Cid, Sara, and Wilhelm Heinrich Holzapfel. "Improved Screening Procedure for Biogenic Amine Production by Lactic Acid Bacteria." *International Journal of Food Microbiology* 53, no. 1 (December 1, 1999): 33–41. https://doi.org/10.1016/S0168-1605(99)00152-X.

Boyden, Steven E., Avanti Desai, Glenn Cruse, Michael L. Young, Hyejeong C. Bolan, Linda M. Scott, A. Robin Eisch, et al. "Vibratory Urticaria Associated with a Missense Variant in ADGRE2." *The New England Journal of Medicine* 374, no. 7 (February 18, 2016): 656–63. https://doi.org/10.1056/NEJMoa1500611.

Branco, Anna Cláudia Calvielli Castelo, Fábio Seiti Yamada Yoshikawa, Anna Julia Pietrobon, and Maria Notomi Sato. "Role of Histamine in Modulating the Immune Response and Inflammation." *Mediators of Inflammation* 2018 (August 27, 2018): e9524075. https://doi.org/10.1155/2018/9524075.

Brew, O., and M. H. F. Sullivan. "The Links between Maternal Histamine Levels and Complications of Human Pregnancy." *Journal of Reproductive Immunology* 72, no. 1 (December 1, 2006): 94–107. https://doi.org/10.1016/j.jri.2006.04.002.

Cao, Suqi, Zicheng Zhang, Lei Liu, Yin Li, Wei Li, Yunling Li, and
    Dingfeng Wu. "Causal Relationships between Atopic
    Dermatitis and Psychiatric Disorders: A Bidirectional Two-
    Sample Mendelian Randomization Study." *BMC Psychiatry*
    24, no. 1 (January 3, 2024): 16. https://doi.org/10.1186/s12888-
    023-05478-1.

Carthy, Elliott, and Tommas Ellender. "Histamine, Neuroinflammation
    and Neurodevelopment: A Review." *Frontiers in Neuroscience*
    15 (July 14, 2021): 680214.
    https://doi.org/10.3389/fnins.2021.680214.

Castellan Baldan, Lissandra, Kyle A. Williams, Jean-Dominique
    Gallezot, Vladimir Pogorelov, Maximiliano Rapanelli, Michael
    Crowley, George M. Anderson, et al. "Histidine Decarboxylase
    Deficiency Causes Tourette Syndrome: Parallel Findings in
    Humans and Mice." *Neuron* 81, no. 1 (January 8, 2014): 77–
    90. https://doi.org/10.1016/j.neuron.2013.10.052.

Chen, Haiwei, Phu-Khat Nwe, Yi Yang, Connor E. Rosen, Agata A.
    Bielecka, Manik Kuchroo, Gary W. Cline, et al. "A Forward
    Chemical Genetic Screen Reveals Gut Microbiota Metabolites
    That Modulate Host Physiology." *Cell* 177, no. 5 (May 16,
    2019): 1217-1231.e18.
    https://doi.org/10.1016/j.cell.2019.03.036.

Chen, Jingshan, Barbara K. Lipska, Nader Halim, Quang D. Ma,
    Mitsuyuki Matsumoto, Samer Melhem, Bhaskar S. Kolachana,
    et al. "Functional Analysis of Genetic Variation in Catechol-O-
    Methyltransferase (COMT): Effects on mRNA, Protein, and
    Enzyme Activity in Postmortem Human Brain." *American
    Journal of Human Genetics* 75, no. 5 (November 2004): 807–
    21. https://doi.org/10.1086/425589.

Chen, Jun, and Xiao-Yong Hu. "Inhibition of Histamine Receptor H3R
    Suppresses Prostate Cancer Growth, Invasion and Increases
    Apoptosis via the AR Pathway." *Oncology Letters* 16, no. 4
    (October 2018): 4921–28.
    https://doi.org/10.3892/ol.2018.9310.

Choi, Yean Jung, So-Yeon Lee, Sung-Ok Kwon, Mi-Jin Kang, Ju-Hee
    Seo, Jisun Yoon, Hyun-Ju Cho, Sungsu Jung, and Soo-Jong
    Hong. "The Association between MTHFR Polymorphism,
    Dietary Methyl Donors, and Childhood Asthma and Atopy."
    Asian Pacific Journal of Allergy and Immunology, January 3,
    2023. https://doi.org/10.12932/AP-300422-1375.

Christ, Pia, Anna Sergeevna Sowa, Oren Froy, and Axel Lorentz. "The
    Circadian Clock Drives Mast Cell Functions in Allergic
    Reactions." *Frontiers in Immunology* 9 (July 6, 2018): 1526.
    https://doi.org/10.3389/fimmu.2018.01526.

Chu, Min, Zhi-Li Huang, Wei-Min Qu, Naomi Eguchi, Ming-Hui Yao,
    and Yoshihiro Urade. "Extracellular Histamine Level in the
    Frontal Cortex Is Positively Correlated with the Amount of
    Wakefulness in Rats." *Neuroscience Research* 49, no. 4
    (August 2004): 417–20.
    https://doi.org/10.1016/j.neures.2004.05.001.

Chung, Bo Young, Sook Young Park, Yun Sun Byun, Jee Hee Son,
    Yong Won Choi, Yong Se Cho, Hye One Kim, and Chun
    Wook Park. "Effect of Different Cooking Methods on
    Histamine Levels in Selected Foods." *Annals of Dermatology*
    29, no. 6 (December 2017): 706–14.
    https://doi.org/10.5021/ad.2017.29.6.706.

De Palma, Giada, Chiko Shimbori, David E. Reed, Yang Yu, Virginia
    Rabbia, Jun Lu, Nestor Jimenez-Vargas, et al. "Histamine
    Production by the Gut Microbiota Induces Visceral
    Hyperalgesia through Histamine 4 Receptor Signaling in
    Mice." *Science Translational Medicine* 14, no. 655 (July 27,
    2022): eabj1895. https://doi.org/10.1126/scitranslmed.abj1895.

Deiteren, A, J G De Man, P A Pelckmans, and B Y De Winter.
    "Histamine H4 Receptors in the Gastrointestinal Tract." *British
    Journal of Pharmacology* 172, no. 5 (March 2015): 1165–78.
    https://doi.org/10.1111/bph.12989.

Dev, Shrabanti, Hiroyuki Mizuguchi, Asish K. Das, Chiyo Matsushita,
    Kazutaka Maeyama, Hayato Umehara, Takayuki Ohtoshi, et al.

"Suppression of Histamine Signaling by Probiotic Lac-B: A Possible Mechanism of Its Anti-Allergic Effect." *Journal of Pharmacological Sciences* 107, no. 2 (2008): 159–66. https://doi.org/10.1254/jphs.08028FP.

Ebbehøj, Niels E., Tove Agner, Erik Zimerson, and Magnus Bruze. "Outbreak of Eczema and Rhinitis in a Group of Office Workers in Greenland." *International Journal of Circumpolar Health* 74 (2015): 27919. https://doi.org/10.3402/ijch.v74.27919.

"Exposure of Children to BPA through Dust and the Association of Urinary BPA and Triclosan with Oxidative Stress in Guangzhou, China - PubMed." Accessed January 11, 2024. https://pubmed.ncbi.nlm.nih.gov/27808329/.

Fujimura, Ririka, Ayano Asada, Misato Aizawa, and Itsuro Kazama. "Cetirizine More Potently Exerts Mast Cell-Stabilizing Property than Diphenhydramine." *Drug Discoveries & Therapeutics* 16, no. 5 (November 20, 2022): 245–50. https://doi.org/10.5582/ddt.2022.01067.

Fukui, Hiroyuki, Hiroyuki Mizuguchi, Hisao Nemoto, Yoshiaki Kitamura, Yoshiki Kashiwada, and Noriaki Takeda. "Histamine H1 Receptor Gene Expression and Drug Action of Antihistamines." *Handbook of Experimental Pharmacology* 241 (2017): 161–69. https://doi.org/10.1007/164_2016_14.

Gao, Feng, and Shanyong Zhang. "Loratadine Alleviates Advanced Glycation End Product-Induced Activation of NLRP3 Inflammasome in Human Chondrocytes." *Drug Design, Development and Therapy* 14 (July 21, 2020): 2899–2908. https://doi.org/10.2147/DDDT.S243512.

Gao, Wei, Yan Zan, Zai-Jie Jim Wang, Xiao-Yu Hu, and Fang Huang. "Quercetin Ameliorates Paclitaxel-Induced Neuropathic Pain by Stabilizing Mast Cells, and Subsequently Blocking PKCε-Dependent Activation of TRPV1." *Acta Pharmacologica Sinica* 37, no. 9 (September 2016): 1166–77. https://doi.org/10.1038/aps.2016.58.

Garai, G., M. T. Dueñas, A. Irastorza, and M. V. Moreno-Arribas. "Biogenic Amine Production by Lactic Acid Bacteria Isolated from Cider." *Letters in Applied Microbiology* 45, no. 5 (November 2007): 473–78. https://doi.org/10.1111/j.1472-765X.2007.02207.x.

García-Martín, Elena, Carmen Martínez, Mercedes Serrador, Hortensia Alonso-Navarro, Pedro Ayuso, Francisco Navacerrada, José A. G. Agúndez, and Félix Javier Jiménez-Jiménez. "Diamine Oxidase Rs10156191 and Rs2052129 Variants Are Associated with the Risk for Migraine." *Headache* 55, no. 2 (February 2015): 276–86. https://doi.org/10.1111/head.12493.

Giannetti, Arianna, Emanuele Filice, Carlo Caffarelli, Giampaolo Ricci, and Andrea Pession. "Mast Cell Activation Disorders." *Medicina* 57, no. 2 (January 30, 2021): 124. https://doi.org/10.3390/medicina57020124.

Gotoh, Koro, Takayuki Masaki, Seiichi Chiba, Keiko Higuchi, Tetsuya Kakuma, Hiroyuki Shimizu, Masatomo Mori, Toshiie Sakata, and Hironobu Yoshimatsu. "Hypothalamic Neuronal Histamine Signaling in the Estrogen Deficiency-Induced Obesity." *Journal of Neurochemistry* 110, no. 6 (September 2009): 1796–1805. https://doi.org/10.1111/j.1471-4159.2009.06272.x.

Graham, Amy C., Rachel M. Temple, and Joshua J. Obar. "Mast Cells and Influenza a Virus: Association with Allergic Responses and Beyond." *Frontiers in Immunology* 6 (2015): 238. https://doi.org/10.3389/fimmu.2015.00238.

Gray, Shelly L., Melissa L. Anderson, Sascha Dublin, Joseph T. Hanlon, Rebecca Hubbard, Rod Walker, Onchee Yu, Paul K. Crane, and Eric B. Larson. "Cumulative Use of Strong Anticholinergics and Incident Dementia: A Prospective Cohort Study." *JAMA Internal Medicine* 175, no. 3 (March 1, 2015): 401–7. https://doi.org/10.1001/jamainternmed.2014.7663.

Griauzdaitė, K., K. Maselis, A. Žvirblienė, A. Vaitkus, D. Jančiauskas, I. Banaitytė-Baleišienė, L. Kupčinskas, and D. Rastenytė.

"Associations between Migraine, Celiac Disease, Non-Celiac Gluten Sensitivity and Activity of Diamine Oxidase." *Medical Hypotheses* 142 (September 2020): 109738. https://doi.org/10.1016/j.mehy.2020.109738.

Guan, Leo C, Xinzhong Dong, and Dustin P Green. "Roles of Mast Cells and Their Interactions with the Trigeminal Nerve in Migraine Headache." *Molecular Pain* 19 (June 1, 2023): 17448069231181358. https://doi.org/10.1177/17448069231181358.

Hagel, Alexander F., Christian M. Layritz, Wolfgang H. Hagel, Hans-Jürgen Hagel, Edith Hagel, Wolfgang Dauth, Jürgen Kressel, et al. "Intravenous Infusion of Ascorbic Acid Decreases Serum Histamine Concentrations in Patients with Allergic and Non-Allergic Diseases." *Naunyn-Schmiedeberg's Archives of Pharmacology* 386, no. 9 (September 2013): 789–93. https://doi.org/10.1007/s00210-013-0880-1.

Han, Eun Su, Joo Yeon Oh, and Hye-Jin Park. "Cordyceps Militaris Extract Suppresses Dextran Sodium Sulfate-Induced Acute Colitis in Mice and Production of Inflammatory Mediators from Macrophages and Mast Cells." *Journal of Ethnopharmacology* 134, no. 3 (April 12, 2011): 703–10. https://doi.org/10.1016/j.jep.2011.01.022.

Hananeh, Wael Mahmoud, Raida Al Rukibat, Shefa Jaradat, and Mohammad Borhan Al-Zghoul. "Exposure Assessment of Bisphenol A by Drinking Coffee from Plastic Cups." *Roczniki Panstwowego Zakladu Higieny* 72, no. 1 (2021): 49–53. https://doi.org/10.32394/rpzh.2021.0146.

Hao, Liuyi, Qian Sun, Wei Zhong, Wenliang Zhang, Xinguo Sun, and Zhanxiang Zhou. "Mitochondria-Targeted Ubiquinone (MitoQ) Enhances Acetaldehyde Clearance by Reversing Alcohol-Induced Posttranslational Modification of Aldehyde Dehydrogenase 2: A Molecular Mechanism of Protection against Alcoholic Liver Disease." *Redox Biology* 14 (April 2018): 626–36. https://doi.org/10.1016/j.redox.2017.11.005.

Hasler, William L., Gintautas Grabauskas, Prashant Singh, and Chung Owyang. "Mast Cell Mediation of Visceral Sensation and Permeability in Irritable Bowel Syndrome." *Neurogastroenterology and Motility* 34, no. 7 (July 2022): e14339. https://doi.org/10.1111/nmo.14339.

He, Gong-Hao, Wen-Ke Cai, Jing-Ru Meng, Xue Ma, Fan Zhang, Jun Lu, and Gui-Li Xu. "Relation of Polymorphism of the Histidine Decarboxylase Gene to Chronic Heart Failure in Han Chinese." *The American Journal of Cardiology* 115, no. 11 (June 1, 2015): 1555–62. https://doi.org/10.1016/j.amjcard.2015.02.062.

Heidari, Abolfazl, Chanakan Tongsook, Reza Najafipour, Luciana Musante, Nasim Vasli, Masoud Garshasbi, Hao Hu, et al. "Mutations in the Histamine N-Methyltransferase Gene, HNMT, Are Associated with Nonsyndromic Autosomal Recessive Intellectual Disability." *Human Molecular Genetics* 24, no. 20 (October 15, 2015): 5697–5710. https://doi.org/10.1093/hmg/ddv286.

Hernandez, Laura M., Elvis Genbo Xu, Hans C. E. Larsson, Rui Tahara, Vimal B. Maisuria, and Nathalie Tufenkji. "Plastic Teabags Release Billions of Microparticles and Nanoparticles into Tea." *Environmental Science & Technology* 53, no. 21 (November 5, 2019): 12300–310. https://doi.org/10.1021/acs.est.9b02540.

Hirasawa, Noriyasu. "Expression of Histidine Decarboxylase and Its Roles in Inflammation." *International Journal of Molecular Sciences* 20, no. 2 (January 16, 2019): 376. https://doi.org/10.3390/ijms20020376.

"Histamine Type-2 Receptor Antagonists (H2 Blockers)." In *LiverTox: Clinical and Research Information on Drug-Induced Liver Injury*. Bethesda (MD): National Institute of Diabetes and Digestive and Kidney Diseases, 2012. http://www.ncbi.nlm.nih.gov/books/NBK547929/.

Hong, X.J., A. Francker, and B. Diamant. "Effects of N-Acetylcysteine on Histamine Release by Sodium Fluoride and Compound 48/80 from Isolated Rat Mast Cells." *International Archives of Allergy and Applied Immunology* 96, no. 4 (September 2, 2009): 338–43. https://doi.org/10.1159/000235518.

Hrubisko, Martin, Radoslav Danis, Martin Huorka, and Martin Wawruch. "Histamine Intolerance—The More We Know the Less We Know. A Review." *Nutrients* 13, no. 7 (June 29, 2021): 2228. https://doi.org/10.3390/nu13072228.

Jarisch, R., D. Weyer, E. Ehlert, C. H. Koch, E. Pinkowski, P. Jung, W. Kähler, et al. "Impact of Oral Vitamin C on Histamine Levels and Seasickness." *Journal of Vestibular Research: Equilibrium & Orientation* 24, no. 4 (2014): 281–88. https://doi.org/10.3233/VES-140509.

Kaag, Sina, and Axel Lorentz. "Effects of Dietary Components on Mast Cells: Possible Use as Nutraceuticals for Allergies?" *Cells* 12, no. 22 (November 10, 2023): 2602. https://doi.org/10.3390/cells12222602.

Kempuraj, D, M Tagen, B P Iliopoulou, A Clemons, M Vasiadi, W Boucher, M House, A Wolfberg, and T C Theoharides. "Luteolin Inhibits Myelin Basic Protein-Induced Human Mast Cell Activation and Mast Cell-Dependent Stimulation of Jurkat T Cells." *British Journal of Pharmacology* 155, no. 7 (December 2008): 1076–84. https://doi.org/10.1038/bjp.2008.356.

Kennedy, Mary Jayne, Jennifer A. Loehle, Angela R. Griffin, Mark A. Doll, Gregory L. Kearns, Janice E. Sullivan, and David W. Hein. "Association of the Histamine N-Methyltransferase C314T (Thr105Ile) Polymorphism with Atopic Dermatitis in Caucasian Children." *Pharmacotherapy* 28, no. 12 (December 2008): 1495–1501. https://doi.org/10.1592/phco.28.12.1495.

Kessler, Aleeza T., and Avais Raja. "Biochemistry, Histidine." In *StatPearls*. Treasure Island (FL): StatPearls Publishing, 2023. http://www.ncbi.nlm.nih.gov/books/NBK538201/.

Kim, Jiyoong, Akiko Ogai, Satoshi Nakatani, Kazuhiko Hashimura, Hideaki Kanzaki, Kazuo Komamura, Masanori Asakura, et al. "Impact of Blockade of Histamine H2 Receptors on Chronic Heart Failure Revealed by Retrospective and Prospective Randomized Studies." *Journal of the American College of Cardiology* 48, no. 7 (October 3, 2006): 1378–84. https://doi.org/10.1016/j.jacc.2006.05.069.

Kim, Kwang H., Jihwan Park, Yejin Cho, Soo Young Cho, Buhyun Lee, Haengdueng Jeong, Yura Lee, et al. "Histamine Signaling Is Essential for Tissue Macrophage Differentiation and Suppression of Bacterial Overgrowth in the Stomach." *Cellular and Molecular Gastroenterology and Hepatology* 15, no. 1 (September 24, 2022): 213–36. https://doi.org/10.1016/j.jcmgh.2022.09.008.

Kimata, M., N. Inagaki, and H. Nagai. "Effects of Luteolin and Other Flavonoids on IgE-Mediated Allergic Reactions." *Planta Medica* 66, no. 1 (February 2000): 25–29. https://doi.org/10.1055/s-2000-11107.

Kishimoto, Yu, Sanki Asakawa, Taiki Sato, Takayuki Takano, Takahisa Nakajyo, Natsumi Mizuno, Ryosuke Segawa, et al. "Induced Histamine Regulates Ni Elution from an Implanted Ni Wire in Mice by Downregulating Neutrophil Migration." *Experimental Dermatology* 26, no. 10 (October 2017): 868–74. https://doi.org/10.1111/exd.13315.

Kline, Jaclyn M., Erica Arriaga-Gomez, Tenzin Yangdon, Beebie Boo, Jasmine Landry, Marietta Saldías-Montivero, Nefeli Neamonitaki, et al. "Repeated Dermal Application of the Common Preservative Methylisothiazolinone Triggers Local Inflammation, T Cell Influx, and Prolonged Mast Cell-Dependent Tactile Sensitivity in Mice." *PLoS ONE* 15, no. 10 (October 26, 2020): e0241218. https://doi.org/10.1371/journal.pone.0241218.

Komericki, Peter, Georg Klein, Norbert Reider, Thomas Hawranek, Tanja Strimitzer, Roland Lang, Bettina Kranzelbinder, and Werner Aberer. "Histamine Intolerance: Lack of Reproducibility of Single Symptoms by Oral Provocation with Histamine: A Randomised, Double-Blind, Placebo-Controlled Cross-over Study." *Wiener Klinische Wochenschrift* 123, no. 1–2 (January 2011): 15–20. https://doi.org/10.1007/s00508-010-1506-y.

Komi, Daniel Elieh Ali, Esmaeil Mortaz, Saeede Amani, Angelica Tiotiu, Gert Folkerts, and Ian M Adcock. "The Role of Mast Cells in IgE-Independent Lung Diseases." *Clinical Reviews in Allergy & Immunology* 58, no. 3 (2020): 377–87. https://doi.org/10.1007/s12016-020-08779-5.

Krell, Tino, José A. Gavira, Félix Velando, Matilde Fernández, Amalia Roca, Elizabet Monteagudo-Cascales, and Miguel A. Matilla. "Histamine: A Bacterial Signal Molecule." *International Journal of Molecular Sciences* 22, no. 12 (June 12, 2021): 6312. https://doi.org/10.3390/ijms22126312.

Kritas, S. K., C. E. Gallenga, C. D Ovidio, G. Ronconi, Al Caraffa, E. Toniato, D. Lauritano, and P. Conti. "Impact of Mold on Mast Cell-Cytokine Immune Response." *Journal of Biological Regulators and Homeostatic Agents* 32, no. 4 (2018): 763–68.

Krušlin, Božo, Davor Tomas, Tihana Džombeta, Marija Milković-Periša, and Monika Ulamec. "Inflammation in Prostatic Hyperplasia and Carcinoma—Basic Scientific Approach." *Frontiers in Oncology* 7 (April 25, 2017): 77. https://doi.org/10.3389/fonc.2017.00077.

Krystel-Whittemore, Melissa, Kottarappat N. Dileepan, and John G. Wood. "Mast Cell: A Multi-Functional Master Cell." *Frontiers in Immunology* 6 (January 6, 2016): 620. https://doi.org/10.3389/fimmu.2015.00620.

Kumar, Sudhir, Marat Khodoun, Eric M. Kettleson, Christopher McKnight, Tiina Reponen, Sergey A. Grinshpun, and Atin Adhikari. "Glyphosate–Rich Air Samples Induce IL–33, TSLP and Generate IL–13 Dependent Airway Inflammation." *Toxicology* 0 (November 5, 2014): 42–51. https://doi.org/10.1016/j.tox.2014.08.008.

Kumari, Asha, D. Dash, and Rashmi Singh. "Lipopolysaccharide (LPS) Exposure Differently Affects Allergic Asthma Exacerbations and Its Amelioration by Intranasal Curcumin in Mice." *Cytokine* 76, no. 2 (December 2015): 334–42. https://doi.org/10.1016/j.cyto.2015.07.022.

Lai, Yuan-Yang, Kung-Chiao Hsieh, Yu-Hsuan Cheng, Keng-Tee Chew, Darian Nguyen, Lalini Ramanathan, and Jerome M Siegel. "Striatal Histamine Mechanism in the Pathogenesis of Restless Legs Syndrome." *Sleep* 43, no. 2 (October 31, 2019): zsz223. https://doi.org/10.1093/sleep/zsz223.

Lama, Adriano, Claudio Pirozzi, Ilenia Severi, Maria Grazia Morgese, Martina Senzacqua, Chiara Annunziata, Federica Comella, et al. "Palmitoylethanolamide Dampens Neuroinflammation and Anxiety-like Behavior in Obese Mice." *Brain, Behavior, and Immunity* 102 (May 2022): 110–23. https://doi.org/10.1016/j.bbi.2022.02.008.

Lee, Jun Ho, Jie Wan Kim, Na Young Ko, Se Hwan Mun, Erk Her, Bo Kyung Kim, Jeung Whan Han, et al. "Curcumin, a Constituent of Curry, Suppresses IgE-Mediated Allergic Response and Mast Cell Activation at the Level of Syk." *Journal of Allergy and Clinical Immunology* 121, no. 5 (May 1, 2008): 1225–31. https://doi.org/10.1016/j.jaci.2007.12.1160.

Lee, Jun-Kyoung, Soyoung Lee, Moon-Chang Baek, Byung-Heon Lee, Hyun-Shik Lee, Taeg Kyu Kwon, Pil-Hoon Park, Tae-Yong Shin, Dongwoo Khang, and Sang-Hyun Kim. "Association between Perfluorooctanoic Acid Exposure and Degranulation of Mast Cells in Allergic Inflammation." *Journal of Applied Toxicology: JAT* 37, no. 5 (May 2017): 554–62. https://doi.org/10.1002/jat.3389.

Lee, Kihwan, Young In Choi, Sang-Taek Im, Sung-Min Hwang, Han-Kyu Lee, Jay-Zoon Im, Yong Ho Kim, Sung Jun Jung, and

Chul-Kyu Park. "Riboflavin Inhibits Histamine-Dependent Itch by Modulating Transient Receptor Potential Vanilloid 1 (TRPV1)." *Frontiers in Molecular Neuroscience* 14 (2021): 643483. https://doi.org/10.3389/fnmol.2021.643483.

Lee, Na Young, Kyung-Sook Chung, Jong Sik Jin, Keuk Soo Bang, Ye-Jin Eom, Chul-Hee Hong, Agung Nugroho, Hee-Jun Park, and Hyo-Jin An. "Effect of Chicoric Acid on Mast Cell-Mediated Allergic Inflammation in Vitro and in Vivo." *Journal of Natural Products* 78, no. 12 (December 24, 2015): 2956–62. https://doi.org/10.1021/acs.jnatprod.5b00668.

Leitner, Roland, Eva Zoernpfenning, and Albert Missbichler. "Evaluation of the Inhibitory Effect of Various Drugs / Active Ingredients on the Activity of Human Diamine Oxidase in Vitro." *Clinical and Translational Allergy* 4, no. S3 (2014): P23. https://doi.org/10.1186/2045-7022-4-S3-P23.

Lertnimitphun, Peeraphong, Wenhui Zhang, Wenwei Fu, Baican Yang, Changwu Zheng, Man Yuan, Hua Zhou, et al. "Safranal Alleviated OVA-Induced Asthma Model and Inhibits Mast Cell Activation." *Frontiers in Immunology* 12 (2021): 585595. https://doi.org/10.3389/fimmu.2021.585595.

Lieberman, Phil. "The Basics of Histamine Biology." *Annals of Allergy, Asthma & Immunology: Official Publication of the American College of Allergy, Asthma, & Immunology* 106, no. 2 Suppl (February 2011): S2-5. https://doi.org/10.1016/j.anai.2010.08.005.

Liu, Hsin-Tzu, Jia-Heng Shie, Sung-Ho Chen, Yu-Syuan Wang, and Hann-Chorng Kuo. "Differences in Mast Cell Infiltration, E-Cadherin, and Zonula Occludens-1 Expression Between Patients With Overactive Bladder and Interstitial Cystitis/Bladder Pain Syndrome." *Urology* 80, no. 1 (July 1, 2012): 225.e13-225.e18. https://doi.org/10.1016/j.urology.2012.01.047.

Liu, Z.-Q., X.-X. Li, S.-Q. Qiu, Y. Yu, M.-G. Li, L.-T. Yang, L.-J. Li, et al. "Vitamin D Contributes to Mast Cell Stabilization."

Allergy 72, no. 8 (2017): 1184–92.
https://doi.org/10.1111/all.13110.

Ma, Jinjin, Yao Nie, Lijie Zhang, and Yan Xu. "Ratio of Histamine-Producing/Non-Histamine-Producing Subgroups of Tetragenococcus Halophilus Determines the Histamine Accumulation during Spontaneous Fermentation of Soy Sauce." *Applied and Environmental Microbiology* 89, no. 3 (n.d.): e01884-22. https://doi.org/10.1128/aem.01884-22.

Maintz, L., C.-F. Yu, E. Rodríguez, H. Baurecht, T. Bieber, T. Illig, S. Weidinger, and Natalija Novak. "Association of Single Nucleotide Polymorphisms in the Diamine Oxidase Gene with Diamine Oxidase Serum Activities." *Allergy* 66, no. 7 (July 2011): 893–902. https://doi.org/10.1111/j.1398-9995.2011.02548.x.

Maintz, Laura, and Natalija Novak. "Histamine and Histamine Intolerance2." *The American Journal of Clinical Nutrition* 85, no. 5 (May 1, 2007): 1185–96.
https://doi.org/10.1093/ajcn/85.5.1185.

Maintz, Laura, Verena Schwarzer, Thomas Bieber, Katrin van der Ven, and Natalija Novak. "Effects of Histamine and Diamine Oxidase Activities on Pregnancy: A Critical Review." *Human Reproduction Update* 14, no. 5 (September 1, 2008): 485–95. https://doi.org/10.1093/humupd/dmn014.

Malhotra, Rakesh. "Understanding Migraine: Potential Role of Neurogenic Inflammation." *Annals of Indian Academy of Neurology* 19, no. 2 (June 2016): 175.
https://doi.org/10.4103/0972-2327.182302.

Malik, Shabana T., Brian R. Birch, David Voegeli, Mandy Fader, Vipul Foria, Alan J. Cooper, Andrew F. Walls, and Bashir A. Lwaleed. "Distribution of Mast Cell Subtypes in Interstitial Cystitis: Implications for Novel Diagnostic and Therapeutic Strategies?" *Journal of Clinical Pathology* 71, no. 9 (September 1, 2018): 840–44. https://doi.org/10.1136/jclinpath-2017-204881.

Maršavelski, Aleksandra, Janez Mavri, Robert Vianello, and Jernej
     Stare. "Why Monoamine Oxidase B Preferably Metabolizes N-
     Methylhistamine over Histamine: Evidence from the
     Multiscale Simulation of the Rate-Limiting Step."
     International Journal of Molecular Sciences 23, no. 3
     (February 8, 2022): 1910.
     https://doi.org/10.3390/ijms23031910.

Martner-Hewes, P. M., I. F. Hunt, N. J. Murphy, M. E. Swendseid, and
     R. H. Settlage. "Vitamin B-6 Nutriture and Plasma Diamine
     Oxidase Activity in Pregnant Hispanic Teenagers." *The
     American Journal of Clinical Nutrition* 44, no. 6 (December
     1986): 907–13. https://doi.org/10.1093/ajcn/44.6.907.

Masini, Emanuela, Danielle Bani, Cosimo Marzocca, Mircea
     Alexandru Mateescu, Pier Francesco Mannaioni, Rodolfo
     Federico, and Bruno Mondovì. "Pea Seedling Histaminase as a
     Novel Therapeutic Approach to Anaphylactic and
     Inflammatory Disorders." *The Scientific World Journal* 7
     (NaN/NaN/NaN): 888–902.
     https://doi.org/10.1100/tsw.2007.139.

McIntosh, Keith, David E. Reed, Theresa Schneider, Frances Dang,
     Ammar H. Keshteli, Giada De Palma, Karen Madsen, Premysl
     Bercik, and Stephen Vanner. "FODMAPs Alter Symptoms and
     the Metabolome of Patients with IBS: A Randomised
     Controlled Trial." *Gut* 66, no. 7 (July 1, 2017): 1241–51.
     https://doi.org/10.1136/gutjnl-2015-311339.

Méndez-Enríquez, Erika, and Jenny Hallgren. "Mast Cells and Their
     Progenitors in Allergic Asthma." *Frontiers in Immunology* 10
     (2019).
     https://www.frontiersin.org/articles/10.3389/fimmu.2019.0082
     1.

Meza-Velázquez, R., F. López-Márquez, S. Espinosa-Padilla, M.
     Rivera-Guillen, J. Ávila-Hernández, and M. Rosales-González.
     "Association of Diamine Oxidase and Histamine N-
     Methyltransferase Polymorphisms with Presence of Migraine
     in a Group of Mexican Mothers of Children with Allergies."

Neurología (English Edition) 32, no. 8 (October 1, 2017): 500–507. https://doi.org/10.1016/j.nrleng.2016.02.012.

Mi, Yan-Ni, Ping-Ping Yan, Rui-Hong Yu, Xue Xiao, Jin Wang, and Lei Cao. "Non-IgE-Mediated Hypersensitivity Induced by Multivitamins Containing Tween-80." *Clinical and Experimental Pharmacology & Physiology* 46, no. 7 (July 2019): 664–75. https://doi.org/10.1111/1440-1681.13089.

"Microbial Patterns in Patients with Histamine Intolerance." *Journal of Physiology and Pharmacology*, 2018. https://doi.org/10.26402/jpp.2018.4.09.

Misaka, Shingen, Yuko Ono, R. Verena Taudte, Eva Hoier, Hiroshi Ogata, Tomoyuki Ono, Jörg König, Hiroshi Watanabe, Martin F. Fromm, and Kenju Shimomura. "Exposure of Fexofenadine, but Not Pseudoephedrine, Is Markedly Decreased by Green Tea Extract in Healthy Volunteers." *Clinical Pharmacology and Therapeutics* 112, no. 3 (September 2022): 627–34. https://doi.org/10.1002/cpt.2682.

Misto, Alessandra, Gustavo Provensi, Valentina Vozella, Maria Beatrice Passani, and Daniele Piomelli. "Mast Cell-Derived Histamine Regulates Liver Ketogenesis via Oleoylethanolamide Signaling." *Cell Metabolism* 29, no. 1 (January 2019): 91-102.e5. https://doi.org/10.1016/j.cmet.2018.09.014.

Mizuguchi, Hiroyuki, Yuko Miyamoto, Takuma Terao, Haruka Yoshida, Wakana Kuroda, Yoshiaki Kitamura, Noriaki Takeda, and Hiroyuki Fukui. "Signaling Pathway of Histamine H1 Receptor-Mediated Histamine H1 Receptor Gene Upregulation Induced by Histamine in U-373 MG Cells." *Current Issues in Molecular Biology* 43, no. 3 (September 24, 2021): 1243–54. https://doi.org/10.3390/cimb43030088.

Monroe, Glen R., Albertien M. van Eerde, Federico Tessadori, Karen J. Duran, Sanne M. C. Savelberg, Johanna C. van Alfen, Paulien A. Terhal, et al. "Identification of Human D Lactate Dehydrogenase Deficiency." *Nature Communications* 10

(April 1, 2019): 1477. https://doi.org/10.1038/s41467-019-09458-6.

Mori, Hiroko, Ken-Ichi Matsuda, Masanaga Yamawaki, and Mitsuhiro Kawata. "Estrogenic Regulation of Histamine Receptor Subtype H1 Expression in the Ventromedial Nucleus of the Hypothalamus in Female Rats." *PLoS ONE* 9, no. 5 (May 7, 2014): e96232. https://doi.org/10.1371/journal.pone.0096232.

Mou, Zhongyu, Yiyan Yang, A. Brantley Hall, and Xiaofang Jiang. "The Taxonomic Distribution of Histamine-Secreting Bacteria in the Human Gut Microbiome." *BMC Genomics* 22, no. 1 (September 26, 2021): 695. https://doi.org/10.1186/s12864-021-08004-3.

Munoz-Cano, R., E. Ainsua-Enrich, I. Torres-Atencio, M. Martin, J. Sánchez-Lopez, J. Bartra, C. Picado, J. Mullol, and A. Valero. "Effects of Rupatadine on Platelet- Activating Factor-Induced Human Mast Cell Degranulation Compared With Desloratadine and Levocetirizine (The MASPAF Study)." *Journal of Investigational Allergology & Clinical Immunology* 27, no. 3 (2017): 161–68. https://doi.org/10.18176/jiaci.0117.

Nakamura, Yuki, Kayoko Ishimaru, Shigenobu Shibata, and Atsuhito Nakao. "Regulation of Plasma Histamine Levels by the Mast Cell Clock and Its Modulation by Stress." *Scientific Reports* 7, no. 1 (January 11, 2017): 39934. https://doi.org/10.1038/srep39934.

Naranjo, Andrea N., Geethani Bandara, Yun Bai, Margery G. Smelkinson, Araceli Tobío, Hirsh D. Komarow, Steven E. Boyden, Daniel L. Kastner, Dean D. Metcalfe, and Ana Olivera. "CRITICAL SIGNALING EVENTS IN THE MECHANOACTIVATION OF HUMAN MAST CELLS VIA P.C492Y-ADGRE2." *The Journal of Investigative Dermatology* 140, no. 11 (November 2020): 2210-2220.e5. https://doi.org/10.1016/j.jid.2020.03.936.

Neree, Armelle Tchoumi, Rodolphe Soret, Lucia Marcocci, Paola Pietrangeli, Nicolas Pilon, and Mircea Alexandru Mateescu.

"Vegetal Diamine Oxidase Alleviates Histamine-Induced Contraction of Colonic Muscles." *Scientific Reports* 10, no. 1 (December 9, 2020): 21563. https://doi.org/10.1038/s41598-020-78134-3.

Nesheim, Nils, Stuart Ellem, Temuujin Dansranjavin, Christina Hagenkötter, Elena Berg, Rupert Schambeck, Hans-Christian Schuppe, et al. "Elevated Seminal Plasma Estradiol and Epigenetic Inactivation of ESR1 and ESR2 Is Associated with CP/CPPS." *Oncotarget* 9, no. 28 (April 13, 2018): 19623–39. https://doi.org/10.18632/oncotarget.24714.

O'Brien, Edmund, Dana C. Dolinoy, and Peter Mancuso. "Bisphenol A at Concentrations Relevant to Human Exposure Enhances Histamine and Cysteinyl Leukotriene Release from Bone Marrow-Derived Mast Cells." *Journal of Immunotoxicology* 11, no. 1 (2014): 84–89. https://doi.org/10.3109/1547691X.2013.800925.

O'Brien, Edmund, Dana C. Dolinoy, and Peter Mancuso. "Perinatal Bisphenol A Exposures Increase Production of Pro-Inflammatory Mediators in Bone Marrow-Derived Mast Cells of Adult Mice." *Journal of Immunotoxicology* 11, no. 3 (2014): 205–12. https://doi.org/10.3109/1547691X.2013.822036.

"Office of Dietary Supplements - Folate." Accessed January 29, 2024. https://ods.od.nih.gov/factsheets/Folate-HealthProfessional/.

Parmar, Ghanshyam, Kilambi Pundarikakshudu, R. Balaraman, and Girish Sailor. "Amelioration of Anaphylaxis, Mast Cell Degranulation and Bronchospasm by Euphorbia Hirta L. Extracts in Experimental Animals." *Beni-Suef University Journal of Basic and Applied Sciences* 7, no. 1 (March 1, 2018): 127–34. https://doi.org/10.1016/j.bjbas.2017.11.001.

Parrella, Edoardo, Vanessa Porrini, Rosa Iorio, Marina Benarese, Annamaria Lanzillotta, Mariana Mota, Mariella Fusco, Paolo Tonin, PierFranco Spano, and Marina Pizzi. "PEA and Luteolin Synergistically Reduce Mast Cell-Mediated Toxicity and Elicit Neuroprotection in Cell-Based Models of Brain

Ischemia." *Brain Research* 1648, no. Pt A (October 1, 2016): 409–17. https://doi.org/10.1016/j.brainres.2016.07.014.

Patel, Raj H., and Shamim S. Mohiuddin. "Biochemistry, Histamine." In *StatPearls*. Treasure Island (FL): StatPearls Publishing, 2023. http://www.ncbi.nlm.nih.gov/books/NBK557790/.

Pattabiraman, Goutham, Ashlee J. Bell-Cohn, Stephen F. Murphy, Daniel J. Mazur, Anthony J. Schaeffer, and Praveen Thumbikat. "Mast Cell Function in Prostate Inflammation, Fibrosis, and Smooth Muscle Cell Dysfunction." *American Journal of Physiology-Renal Physiology* 321, no. 4 (October 2021): F466–79. https://doi.org/10.1152/ajprenal.00116.2021.

Peng, Xueqian, Linlin Yang, Zixuan Liu, Siyi Lou, Shiliu Mei, Meiling Li, Zhong Chen, and Haitao Zhang. "Structural Basis for Recognition of Antihistamine Drug by Human Histamine Receptor." *Nature Communications* 13, no. 1 (October 15, 2022): 6105. https://doi.org/10.1038/s41467-022-33880-y.

Perna, Eluisa, Javier Aguilera-Lizarraga, Morgane V. Florens, Piyush Jain, Stavroula A. Theofanous, Nikita Hanning, Joris G. De Man, et al. "Effect of Resolvins on Sensitisation of TRPV1 and Visceral Hypersensitivity in IBS." *Gut* 70, no. 7 (July 1, 2021): 1275–86. https://doi.org/10.1136/gutjnl-2020-321530.

Pessione, Enrica, and Simona Cirrincione. "Bioactive Molecules Released in Food by Lactic Acid Bacteria: Encrypted Peptides and Biogenic Amines." *Frontiers in Microbiology* 7 (June 9, 2016): 876. https://doi.org/10.3389/fmicb.2016.00876.

Pham, Linh, Leonardo Baiocchi, Lindsey Kennedy, Keisaku Sato, Vik Meadows, Fanyin Meng, Chiung-Kuei Huang, et al. "The Interplay between Mast Cells, Pineal Gland, and Circadian Rhythm: Links between Histamine, Melatonin, and Inflammatory Mediators." *Journal of Pineal Research* 70, no. 2 (March 2021): e12699. https://doi.org/10.1111/jpi.12699.

Piliponsky, Adrian M., Manasa Acharya, and Nicholas J. Shubin. "Mast Cells in Viral, Bacterial, and Fungal Infection Immunity." *International Journal of Molecular Sciences* 20,

no. 12 (June 12, 2019): 2851.
https://doi.org/10.3390/ijms20122851.

Pohanka, Miroslav. "D-Lactic Acid as a Metabolite: Toxicology, Diagnosis, and Detection." *BioMed Research International* 2020 (June 17, 2020): 3419034. https://doi.org/10.1155/2020/3419034.

Prakash, Anupam, Angel Jemima, Sugitharini Vasanth, Gomathi Nagarajan, and Berla Elden. "Effect of Ocimum Tenuiflorum Linn Extract on Histamine Mediated Allergic Inflammation in Human Mast Cells." *Journal of Biologically Active Products from Nature* 7 (February 17, 2017): 1–8. https://doi.org/10.1080/22311866.2016.1275983.

Qian, Hong, Chang Shu, Ling Xiao, and Gaohua Wang. "Histamine and Histamine Receptors: Roles in Major Depressive Disorder." *Frontiers in Psychiatry* 13 (September 23, 2022): 825591. https://doi.org/10.3389/fpsyt.2022.825591.

Rahimzadeh, Ghazal, Abdullatif Tay, Nikolaj Travica, Kathleen Lacy, Shady Mohamed, Darius Nahavandi, Paweł Pławiak, Mohammadreza Chalak Qazani, and Houshyar Asadi. "Nutritional and Behavioral Countermeasures as Medication Approaches to Relieve Motion Sickness: A Comprehensive Review." *Nutrients* 15, no. 6 (January 2023): 1320. https://doi.org/10.3390/nu15061320.

Raje, Nikita, Carrie A. Vyhlidal, Hongying Dai, and Bridgette L. Jones. "Genetic Variation within the Histamine Pathway among Patients with Asthma." *The Journal of Asthma : Official Journal of the Association for the Care of Asthma* 52, no. 4 (May 2015): 353–62. https://doi.org/10.3109/02770903.2014.973501.

Reddy, Yugandhar P., Santosh Tiwari, Lomas K. Tomar, Nalini Desai, and Varun Kumar Sharma. "Fluoride-Induced Expression of Neuroinflammatory Markers and Neurophysiological Regulation in the Brain of Wistar Rat Model." *Biological*

Trace Element Research 199, no. 7 (July 2021): 2621–26.
https://doi.org/10.1007/s12011-020-02362-x.

Regecová, Ivana, Boris Semjon, Pavlina Jevinová, Peter Očenáš, Jana
Výrostková, Lucia Šuľáková, Erika Nosková, Slavomír
Marcinčák, and Martin Bartkovský. "Detection of Microbiota
during the Fermentation Process of Wine in Relation to the
Biogenic Amine Content." *Foods* 11, no. 19 (October 2, 2022):
3061. https://doi.org/10.3390/foods11193061.

Rock, R. Bryan, Genya Gekker, Shuxian Hu, Wen S. Sheng, Maxim
Cheeran, James R. Lokensgard, and Phillip K. Peterson. "Role
of Microglia in Central Nervous System Infections." *Clinical
Microbiology Reviews* 17, no. 4 (October 2004): 942–64.
https://doi.org/10.1128/CMR.17.4.942-964.2004.

Romero, Steven A., Matthew R. Ely, Dylan C. Sieck, Meredith J.
Luttrell, Tahisha M. Buck, Jordan M. Kono, Adam J.
Branscum, and John R. Halliwill. "Effect of Antioxidants on
Histamine Receptor Activation and Sustained Post-Exercise
Vasodilatation in Humans." *Experimental Physiology* 100, no.
4 (April 1, 2015): 435–49. https://doi.org/10.1113/EP085030.

Romero, Steven A., Jennifer L. McCord, Matthew R. Ely, Dylan C.
Sieck, Tahisha M. Buck, Meredith J. Luttrell, David A.
MacLean, and John R. Halliwill. "Mast Cell Degranulation and
de Novo Histamine Formation Contribute to Sustained
Postexercise Vasodilation in Humans." *Journal of Applied
Physiology* 122, no. 3 (March 1, 2017): 603–10.
https://doi.org/10.1152/japplphysiol.00633.2016.

Roy, Saptarshi, Chalatip Chompunud Na Ayudhya, Monica Thapaliya,
Vishwa Deepak, and Hydar Ali. "Multifaceted MRGPRX2:
New Insight into the Role of Mast Cells in Health and
Disease." *The Journal of Allergy and Clinical Immunology*
148, no. 2 (August 2021): 293–308.
https://doi.org/10.1016/j.jaci.2021.03.049.

Sánchez-Pérez, Sònia, Oriol Comas-Basté, Judit Costa-Catala, Irache
Iduriaga-Platero, M. Teresa Veciana-Nogués, M. Carmen

Vidal-Carou, and M. Luz Latorre-Moratalla. "The Rate of Histamine Degradation by Diamine Oxidase Is Compromised by Other Biogenic Amines." *Frontiers in Nutrition* 9 (May 25, 2022): 897028. https://doi.org/10.3389/fnut.2022.897028.

———. "The Rate of Histamine Degradation by Diamine Oxidase Is Compromised by Other Biogenic Amines." *Frontiers in Nutrition* 9 (May 25, 2022): 897028. https://doi.org/10.3389/fnut.2022.897028.

Sánchez-Pérez, Sònia, Oriol Comas-Basté, Adriana Duelo, M. Teresa Veciana-Nogués, Mercedes Berlanga, M. Luz Latorre-Moratalla, and M. Carmen Vidal-Carou. "Intestinal Dysbiosis in Patients with Histamine Intolerance." *Nutrients* 14, no. 9 (April 23, 2022): 1774. https://doi.org/10.3390/nu14091774.

Sato, Takahiko, Masato Taguchi, Hisamitsu Nagase, Hideaki Kito, and Miki Niikawa. "Augmentation of Allergic Reactions by Several Pesticides." *Toxicology* 126, no. 1 (February 20, 1998): 41–53. https://doi.org/10.1016/S0300-483X(97)00184-4.

Savvaides, Tina, Jeremy P. Koelmel, Yakun Zhou, Elizabeth Z. Lin, Paul Stelben, Juan J. Aristizabal-Henao, John A. Bowden, and Krystal J. Godri Pollitt. "Prevalence and Implications of Per- and Polyfluoroalkyl Substances (PFAS) in Settled Dust." *Current Environmental Health Reports* 8, no. 4 (December 1, 2021): 323–35. https://doi.org/10.1007/s40572-021-00326-4.

Schaubschläger, W. W., W. M. Becker, U. Schade, P. Zabel, and M. Schlaak. "Release of Mediators from Human Gastric Mucosa and Blood in Adverse Reactions to Benzoate." *International Archives of Allergy and Applied Immunology* 96, no. 2 (1991): 97–101. https://doi.org/10.1159/000235478.

Schink, M., P. C. Konturek, E. Tietz, W. Dieterich, T. C. Pinzer, S. Wirtz, M. F. Neurath, and Y. Zopf. "Microbial Patterns in Patients with Histamine Intolerance." *Journal of Physiology and Pharmacology: An Official Journal of the Polish Physiological Society* 69, no. 4 (August 2018). https://doi.org/10.26402/jpp.2018.4.09.

Schirmer, Bastian, and Detlef Neumann. "The Function of the Histamine H4 Receptor in Inflammatory and Inflammation-Associated Diseases of the Gut." *International Journal of Molecular Sciences* 22, no. 11 (June 6, 2021): 6116. https://doi.org/10.3390/ijms22116116.

Schnedl, Wolfgang J., Sonja Lackner, Dietmar Enko, Michael Schenk, Sandra J. Holasek, and Harald Mangge. "Evaluation of Symptoms and Symptom Combinations in Histamine Intolerance." *Intestinal Research* 17, no. 3 (July 2019): 427–33. https://doi.org/10.5217/ir.2018.00152.

Schnedl, Wolfgang J., Sonja Lackner, Dietmar Enko, Michael Schenk, Harald Mangge, and Sandra J. Holasek. "Non-Celiac Gluten Sensitivity: People without Celiac Disease Avoiding Gluten-Is It Due to Histamine Intolerance?" *Inflammation Research: Official Journal of the European Histamine Research Society ... [et Al.]* 67, no. 4 (April 2018): 279–84. https://doi.org/10.1007/s00011-017-1117-4.

Schnedl, Wolfgang J., Michael Schenk, Sonja Lackner, Dietmar Enko, Harald Mangge, and Florian Forster. "Diamine Oxidase Supplementation Improves Symptoms in Patients with Histamine Intolerance." *Food Science and Biotechnology* 28, no. 6 (May 24, 2019): 1779–84. https://doi.org/10.1007/s10068-019-00627-3.

Semerjian, Lucy, Najla Alawadhi, and Khulud Nazer. "Detection of Bisphenol A in Thermal Paper Receipts and Assessment of Human Exposure: A Case Study from Sharjah, United Arab Emirates." *PLOS ONE* 18, no. 3 (March 28, 2023): e0283675. https://doi.org/10.1371/journal.pone.0283675.

Shahriar, Masum, Hiroyuki Mizuguchi, Kazutaka Maeyama, Yoshiaki Kitamura, Naoki Orimoto, Shuhei Horio, Hayato Umehara, Masashi Hattori, Noriaki Takeda, and Hiroyuki Fukui. "Suplatast Tosilate Inhibits Histamine Signaling by Direct and Indirect Down-Regulation of Histamine H1 Receptor Gene Expression through Suppression of Histidine Decarboxylase and IL-4 Gene Transcriptions1." *The Journal of Immunology*

183, no. 3 (August 1, 2009): 2133–41.
https://doi.org/10.4049/jimmunol.0901058.

Shan, Ling, Xin-Rui Qi, Rawien Balesar, Dick F. Swaab, and Ai-Min
Bao. "Unaltered Histaminergic System in Depression: A
Postmortem Study." *Journal of Affective Disorders* 146, no. 2
(April 5, 2013): 220–23.
https://doi.org/10.1016/j.jad.2012.09.008.

Shirley, Devon, Cody McHale, and Gregorio Gomez. "Resveratrol
Preferentially Inhibits IgE-Dependent PGD2 Biosynthesis but
Enhances TNF Production from Human Skin Mast Cells."
Biochimica et Biophysica Acta 1860, no. 4 (April 2016): 678–
85. https://doi.org/10.1016/j.bbagen.2016.01.006.

Shulpekova, Yulia O., Vladimir M. Nechaev, Irina R. Popova, Tatiana
A. Deeva, Arthur T. Kopylov, Kristina A. Malsagova, Anna L.
Kaysheva, and Vladimir T. Ivashkin. "Food Intolerance: The
Role of Histamine." *Nutrients* 13, no. 9 (September 15, 2021):
3207. https://doi.org/10.3390/nu13093207.

"Snapshot." Accessed December 22, 2023.
https://ods.od.nih.gov/factsheets/VitaminB6-
HealthProfessional/.

Son, Jee Hee, Bo Young Chung, Hye One Kim, and Chun Wook Park.
"A Histamine-Free Diet Is Helpful for Treatment of Adult
Patients with Chronic Spontaneous Urticaria." *Annals of
Dermatology* 30, no. 2 (April 2018): 164–72.
https://doi.org/10.5021/ad.2018.30.2.164.

Spanos, C., X. Pang, K. Ligris, R. Letourneau, L. Alferes, N.
Alexacos, G. R. Sant, and T. C. Theoharides. "Stress-Induced
Bladder Mast Cell Activation: Implications for Interstitial
Cystitis." *The Journal of Urology* 157, no. 2 (February 1997):
669–72.

Stevenson, Jim, Edmund Sonuga-Barke, Donna McCann, Kate
Grimshaw, Karen M. Parker, Matthew J. Rose-Zerilli, John W.
Holloway, and John O. Warner. "The Role of Histamine
Degradation Gene Polymorphisms in Moderating the Effects of

Food Additives on Children's ADHD Symptoms." *American Journal of Psychiatry* 167, no. 9 (September 2010): 1108–15. https://doi.org/10.1176/appi.ajp.2010.09101529.

Strawn, Jeffrey R., Laura Geracioti, Neil Rajdev, Kelly Clemenza, and Amir Levine. "Pharmacotherapy for Generalized Anxiety Disorder in Adults and Pediatric Patients: An Evidence-Based Treatment Review." *Expert Opinion on Pharmacotherapy* 19, no. 10 (July 2018): 1057–70. https://doi.org/10.1080/14656566.2018.1491966.

Stromberga, Zane, Russ Chess-Williams, and Christian Moro. "Histamine Modulation of Urinary Bladder Urothelium, Lamina Propria and Detrusor Contractile Activity via H1 and H2 Receptors." *Scientific Reports* 9 (March 7, 2019): 3899. https://doi.org/10.1038/s41598-019-40384-1.

Stuivenberg, Gerrit, Brendan Daisley, Polycronis Akouris, and Gregor Reid. "In Vitro Assessment of Histamine and Lactate Production by a Multi-Strain Synbiotic." *Journal of Food Science and Technology* 59, no. 9 (September 2022): 3419–27. https://doi.org/10.1007/s13197-021-05327-7.

Tachibana, Hirofumi, Yoshinori Fujimura, Yusuke Hasegawa, Satomi Yano, and Koji Yamada. "The Downregulation of Mast Cell Activation Through the Suppression of the High-Affinity IgE Receptor Expression by Green Tea Catechin Egcg." In *Animal Cell Technology: Basic & Applied Aspects*, edited by Masamichi Kamihira, Yoshinori Katakura, and Akira Ito, 301– 6. Animal Cell Technology: Basic & Applied Aspects. Dordrecht: Springer Netherlands, 2010. https://doi.org/10.1007/978-90-481-3892-0_50.

Takahashi, Kazumi, Jian-Sheng Lin, and Kazuya Sakai. "Neuronal Activity of Histaminergic Tuberomammillary Neurons During Wake–Sleep States in the Mouse." *The Journal of Neuroscience* 26, no. 40 (October 4, 2006): 10292–98. https://doi.org/10.1523/JNEUROSCI.2341-06.2006.

Talkington, Jeffrey, and Steven P. Nickell. "Borrelia Burgdorferi Spirochetes Induce Mast Cell Activation and Cytokine Release." *Infection and Immunity* 67, no. 3 (March 1999): 1107–15.

Talwar, Manjit, Amrit Tewari, H. S. Chawla, Vinod Sachdev, and Suresh Sharma. "Fluoride Concentration in Saliva Following Professional Topical Application of 2% Sodium Fluoride Solution." *Contemporary Clinical Dentistry* 10, no. 3 (2019): 423–27. https://doi.org/10.4103/ccd.ccd_681_18.

Tang, Tao, Tianyu Shi, Kun Qian, Pingliang Li, Jianqiang Li, and Yongsong Cao. "Determination of Biogenic Amines in Beer with Pre-Column Derivatization by High Performance Liquid Chromatography." *Journal of Chromatography. B, Analytical Technologies in the Biomedical and Life Sciences* 877, no. 5–6 (February 15, 2009): 507–12. https://doi.org/10.1016/j.jchromb.2008.12.064.

Tao, Ran, Zhicheng Fu, and Lijun Xiao. "Chronic Food Antigen-Specific IgG-Mediated Hypersensitivity Reaction as A Risk Factor for Adolescent Depressive Disorder." *Genomics, Proteomics & Bioinformatics* 17, no. 2 (April 2019): 183–89. https://doi.org/10.1016/j.gpb.2019.05.002.

Theoharides, T C, I Tsilioni, A B Patel, and R Doyle. "Atopic Diseases and Inflammation of the Brain in the Pathogenesis of Autism Spectrum Disorders." *Translational Psychiatry* 6, no. 6 (June 2016): e844. https://doi.org/10.1038/tp.2016.77.

Thomas, Carissa M., Teresa Hong, Jan Peter van Pijkeren, Peera Hemarajata, Dan V. Trinh, Weidong Hu, Robert A. Britton, Markus Kalkum, and James Versalovic. "Histamine Derived from Probiotic Lactobacillus Reuteri Suppresses TNF via Modulation of PKA and ERK Signaling." *PloS One* 7, no. 2 (2012): e31951. https://doi.org/10.1371/journal.pone.0031951.

Tu, Longlong, Zengbing Lu, Karolina Dieser, Christina Schmitt, Sze Wa Chan, Man P. Ngan, Paul L. R. Andrews, Eugene Nalivaiko, and John A. Rudd. "Brain Activation by H1

Antihistamines Challenges Conventional View of Their
Mechanism of Action in Motion Sickness: A Behavioral, c-Fos
and Physiological Study in Suncus Murinus (House Musk
Shrew)." *Frontiers in Physiology* 8 (June 14, 2017): 412.
https://doi.org/10.3389/fphys.2017.00412.

Uranga, José Antonio, Vicente Martínez, and Raquel Abalo. "Mast
Cell Regulation and Irritable Bowel Syndrome: Effects of Food
Components with Potential Nutraceutical Use." *Molecules* 25,
no. 18 (January 2020): 4314.
https://doi.org/10.3390/molecules25184314.

Webb, Lauren M., and Elia D. Tait Wojno. "The Role of Rare Innate
Immune Cells in Type 2 Immune Activation against Parasitic
Helminths." *Parasitology* 144, no. 10 (September 2017): 1288–
1301. https://doi.org/10.1017/S0031182017000488.

Weinstock, Leonard B., Arthur S. Walters, Jill B. Brook, Zahid
Kaleem, Lawrence B. Afrin, and Gerhard J. Molderings.
"Restless Legs Syndrome Is Associated with Mast Cell
Activation Syndrome." *Journal of Clinical Sleep Medicine* 16,
no. 3 (n.d.): 401–8. https://doi.org/10.5664/jcsm.8216.

Wilzopolski, Jenny, Manfred Kietzmann, Santosh K. Mishra, Holger
Stark, Wolfgang Bäumer, and Kristine Rossbach. "TRPV1 and
TRPA1 Channels Are Both Involved Downstream of
Histamine-Induced Itch." *Biomolecules* 11, no. 8 (August 6,
2021): 1166. https://doi.org/10.3390/biom11081166.

Winther, L, Cm Reimert, Ps Skov, L Kærgaard Poulsen, and L
Moseholm. "Basophil Histamine Release, IgE, Eosinophil
Counts, ECP, and EPX Are Related to the Severity of
Symptoms in Seasonal Allergic Rhinitis." *Allergy* 54, no. 5
(1999): 436–45. https://doi.org/10.1034/j.1398-
9995.1999.00910.x.

Worm, Jacob, Katrine Falkenberg, and Jes Olesen. "Histamine and
Migraine Revisited: Mechanisms and Possible Drug Targets."
The Journal of Headache and Pain 20, no. 1 (March 25, 2019):
30. https://doi.org/10.1186/s10194-019-0984-1.

Xanthos, Dimitris N, Simon Gaderer, Ruth Drdla, Erin Nuro, Anastasia Abramova, Wilfried Ellmeier, and Jürgen Sandkühler. "Central Nervous System Mast Cells in Peripheral Inflammatory Nociception." *Molecular Pain* 7 (June 3, 2011): 42. https://doi.org/10.1186/1744-8069-7-42.

Xu, Jiawen, Xiang Zhang, Qingqing Qian, Yiwei Wang, Hongquan Dong, Nana Li, Yanning Qian, and Wenjie Jin. "Histamine Upregulates the Expression of Histamine Receptors and Increases the Neuroprotective Effect of Astrocytes." *Journal of Neuroinflammation* 15 (2018). https://doi.org/10.1186/s12974-018-1068-x.

Yacoub, Mona-Rita, Giuseppe A. Ramirez, Alvise Berti, Giuseppe Mercurio, Daniela Breda, Nicoletta Saporiti, Samuele Burastero, Lorenzo Dagna, and Giselda Colombo. "Diamine Oxidase Supplementation in Chronic Spontaneous Urticaria: A Randomized, Double-Blind Placebo-Controlled Study." *International Archives of Allergy and Immunology* 176, no. 3–4 (2018): 268–71. https://doi.org/10.1159/000488142.

Yamauchi, Kohei, and Masahito Ogasawara. "The Role of Histamine in the Pathophysiology of Asthma and the Clinical Efficacy of Antihistamines in Asthma Therapy." *International Journal of Molecular Sciences* 20, no. 7 (April 8, 2019): 1733. https://doi.org/10.3390/ijms20071733.

Yang, Ming-Tao, Chia-Chun Chen, Wang-Tso Lee, Jao-Shwann Liang, Wen-Mei Fu, and Yao-Hsu Yang. "Attention-Deficit/Hyperactivity Disorder-Related Symptoms Improved with Allergic Rhinitis Treatment in Children." *American Journal of Rhinology & Allergy* 30, no. 3 (May 2016): 209–14. https://doi.org/10.2500/ajra.2016.30.4301.

Yang, Niu-Niu, Hao Shi, Guang Yu, Chang-Ming Wang, Chan Zhu, Yan Yang, Xiao-Lin Yuan, et al. "Osthole Inhibits Histamine-Dependent Itch via Modulating TRPV1 Activity." *Scientific Reports* 6 (May 10, 2016): 25657. https://doi.org/10.1038/srep25657.

Yin, Na, Hongwei Yang, Wei Yao, and Guanghong Ding. "A
    Mathematical Model of Histamine-Mediated Neural Activation
    during Acupuncture." *Biomechanics and Modeling in
    Mechanobiology* 16, no. 5 (October 2017): 1659–68.
    https://doi.org/10.1007/s10237-017-0911-9.

Yoshikawa, Takeo, Tadaho Nakamura, and Kazuhiko Yanai.
    "Histamine N-Methyltransferase in the Brain." *International
    Journal of Molecular Sciences* 20, no. 3 (February 10, 2019):
    737. https://doi.org/10.3390/ijms20030737.

———. "Histamine N-Methyltransferase in the Brain." *International
    Journal of Molecular Sciences* 20, no. 3 (February 10, 2019):
    737. https://doi.org/10.3390/ijms20030737.

Zaitsu, Masafumi, Shin-Ichiro Narita, K. Chad Lambert, James J.
    Grady, D. Mark Estes, Edward M. Curran, Edward G. Brooks,
    Cheryl S. Watson, Randall M. Goldblum, and Terumi Midoro-
    Horiuti. "Estradiol Activates Mast Cells via a Non-Genomic
    Estrogen Receptor-α and Calcium Influx." *Molecular
    Immunology* 44, no. 8 (March 2007): 1977–85.
    https://doi.org/10.1016/j.molimm.2006.09.030.

Zaki, Muhammad, Philip E. Coudron, Robert W. McCuen, Leslie
    Harrington, Shijian Chu, and Mitchell L. Schubert. "H. Pylori
    Acutely Inhibits Gastric Secretion by Activating CGRP
    Sensory Neurons Coupled to Stimulation of Somatostatin and
    Inhibition of Histamine Secretion." *American Journal of
    Physiology. Gastrointestinal and Liver Physiology* 304, no. 8
    (April 15, 2013): G715-722.
    https://doi.org/10.1152/ajpgi.00187.2012.

Zhang, Li-Li, Jun-Qin Wang, Rui-Rui Qi, Lei-Lei Pan, Min Li, and
    Yi-Ling Cai. "Motion Sickness: Current Knowledge and
    Recent Advance." *CNS Neuroscience & Therapeutics* 22, no. 1
    (October 9, 2015): 15–24. https://doi.org/10.1111/cns.12468.

Zhang, Xiang, Hongquan Dong, Nana Li, Susu Zhang, Jie Sun, Shu
    Zhang, and Yanning Qian. "Activated Brain Mast Cells
    Contribute to Postoperative Cognitive Dysfunction by Evoking

Microglia Activation and Neuronal Apoptosis." *Journal of Neuroinflammation* 13 (May 31, 2016): 127. https://doi.org/10.1186/s12974-016-0592-9.

Zhang, Xiao-Yang, Shi-Yu Peng, Li-Ping Shen, Qian-Xing Zhuang, Bin Li, Shu-Tao Xie, Qian-Xiao Li, et al. "Targeting Presynaptic H3 Heteroreceptor in Nucleus Accumbens to Improve Anxiety and Obsessive-Compulsive-like Behaviors." *Proceedings of the National Academy of Sciences of the United States of America* 117, no. 50 (December 15, 2020): 32155–64. https://doi.org/10.1073/pnas.2008456117.

Zierau, Oliver, Ana C. Zenclussen, and Federico Jensen. "Role of Female Sex Hormones, Estradiol and Progesterone, in Mast Cell Behavior." *Frontiers in Immunology* 3 (June 19, 2012). https://doi.org/10.3389/fimmu.2012.00169.

Zimatkin, S. M., and O. V. Anichtchik. "Alcohol-Histamine Interactions." *Alcohol and Alcoholism (Oxford, Oxfordshire)* 34, no. 2 (1999): 141–47. https://doi.org/10.1093/alcalc/34.2.141.